NEGOTIATING SEXUAL AND REPRODUCTIVE JUSTICE

Negotiating Sexual and Reproductive Justice

Voices from the Margins

Edited by

T.K. SUNDARI RAVINDRAN
RENU KHANNA
SUBHA SRI B.

CommonHealth
COALITION FOR REPRODUCTIVE
HEALTH AND SAFE ABORTION, INDIA

MANOHAR
2026

First published 2026
First eBook edition 2026

ISBN 978-93-6080-152-6 (hardbound)
ISBN 978-93-6080-206-6 (ebook)

Published by

Ajay Kumar Jain *for*
Manohar Publishers & Distributors
4753/23 Ansari Road, Daryaganj
New Delhi 110 002

Cover design by Manoj Kumar

Typeset by Kohli Print, Delhi 110 051

Printed and bound in India

Contents

Acknowledgements

This book is based on a qualitative study on the reproductive histories of marginalized women. First and foremost, we would like to thank all the women in the five field areas who trusted us with their life stories. They were generous with their time and their reflections.

Thanks also to

- CommonHealth members for welcoming the idea of documenting the life histories of women amongst whom they work.
- The teams of five organizations that undertook the study.
- Members of the Ethics Committee for their review of the study protocol.
- Swati Shinde, the Coordinator and Programme Manager of CommonHealth, for all her backup support.
- Sabitha for her help in copy editing this manuscript.
- Anuradha Bhasin, for her editorial support, which helped even out the different writing styles of the authors.
- Madhumita Das, who contributed to the development of the methodology.
- To all the reviewers—anonymous reviewers of this manuscript, and Sanjeeta Gawri of CommonHealth, for reviewing various versions of the study outputs.

We are happy to share with a broader audience the insights we gained on the challenges to sexual and reproductive justice experienced by many women in this country.

THE EDITORS

CHAPTER 1

Introduction: Setting the Context for Sharing Our Stories

T.K. SUNDARI RAVINDRAN,
RENU KHANNA and
SUBHA SRI B.

BACKGROUND

> 'Until the lions have their historians, tales of the hunt shall always glorify the hunter'—so goes an African proverb, to describe how dominant groups control the historical narrative.

Feminist standpoint theory puts forth a similar idea when taking the position that knowledge is always socially situated and most often reflects the standpoint of the more powerful, those at the top rungs of the social hierarchy. This often results in epistemic injustice, whereby the knowledge base excludes knowledge about entire groups of people (Fricker 2007).

The literature on public health in India illustrates how what counts as evidence in an academic discipline may obliterate the experiences of entire population groups, masking gross health inequalities. A synthesis of evidence on health inequities in India (Ravindran & Gaitonde 2018) highlighted the sparse evidence on the health concerns of structurally excluded, or 'marginalized' populations such as Dalits, Adivasis, Lesbian, Gay, Bisexual, Transgender, Intersex or Queer (LGBTIQ) and persons with disability, among others, contributing to further accentuation of health inequities owing to a lack of evidence for policy and programmatic action on the unmet health needs of structurally excluded populations. Marginalization refers to being distanced from power and resources that enables economic, social and political self-determination. Different population groups may be identified as marginalized in different settings, depending on the historical, socio-economic and political contexts (Daniel & Linder 2002).

The sparsity of evidence on marginalized groups is reflected in the body of knowledge on sexual and reproductive health and rights (SRHR) in India. Important components of sexual and reproductive health and rights include: access to comprehensive sexuality education and sexual and reproductive health services; having violence-free and pleasurable sexual relations and making decisions related to whether, when and who to be sexually active with, whether, when and who to marry and whether, when and how many children to have United Nations Population Fund (UNFPA) 2019.

In a recent review of 481 studies published since 2011 on sexual and reproductive health,[1] 74 per cent (356) did not mention the social locations of the study participants. Of the 26 per cent (125 studies) that examined the prevalence of health problems or health-seeking behaviour by social location, e.g., geographic location, age, caste/ethnicity, economic position, minority status and educational status, the vast majority (88) merely noted that the association of less advantageous social locations (i.e., low socio-economic status or lack of formal schooling) with health outcomes was a predictor of a health outcome. Only 37, or barely 8 per cent, of the articles reviewed were about specific marginalized population groups such as Scheduled Castes or Tribes, urban slum dwellers or sex workers; 12 of these were qualitative studies presenting the perspectives and lived realities of these marginalized groups.

Studies based on the analysis of large scale national surveys such as the National Family Health Surveys confirm that women from the lowest and low wealth quintiles, or belonging to the Scheduled Castes and Scheduled Tribes, or with no formal schooling have lower rates of utilization of antenatal and postnatal care, skilled birth attendance, or institutional delivery (Ram et al. 2011; Singh et al. 2012; Kumar & Singh 2016; Sridharan et al. 2017; Singh et al. 2019; Kumar et al. 2019; Paul et al. 2019; Mohanty et al. 2020; Yadav et al. 2020; Ali et al. 2021; Singh et al. 2021; Yadav et al. 2021; Bango & Ghosh 2022). According to two systematic reviews, when women from these groups do reach a health facility to deliver, they are more likely than their more privileged counterparts to receive abusive and disrespectful care (Ansari & Yeravdekar 2021; Jungari et al. 2021). Women from economically and socially marginalized households also have a higher probability of experiencing maternal death (Tripathi & Mishra 2017; Rane et al. 2019; Khanna et al. 2021); serious complications (Singhal et al. 2018; Kumar & Tewari 2018; Panda et al. 2019), infectious diseases including HIV (Sharma et al. 2021; Kotdawala et al. 2022; Tanwar et al. 2022 and others), mental health problems (for example, Raghavan et al. 2021; Aslam et al. 2022; George et al. 2022) or long-term morbidity (Swain et al. 2020) during pregnancy, child delivery or postpartum.

Among adolescents and young people (15-24 years), analysis of NFHS-4 data (2015-16) indicates that the unmet need for contraception was higher among women with a lower level of education and from low-income households (Sharma et al. 2021). Contraceptive prevalence rates among married adolescent women (15-19 years) were significantly lower for those from rural settings, without formal education, from households belonging to the poorest wealth quintile, and without exposure to family planning messages (Singh et al. 2021). A review of the research in India on knowledge, attitude, practices, and life skills related to sexual and reproductive health among adolescent girls indicates that young women from families below the poverty line and those from backward class communities are unaware of contraceptives and contraceptive practices (Parida et al. 2021). A study on the perceptions of the health needs of urban disadvantaged adolescent girls (living in New Delhi) highlighted their fear of gender-based violence from boys in the neighbourhood, their lack of social networks because of restrictions on their mobility, and the embarrassment and lack of confidentiality they experience while accessing health services, which adversely impact their sexual and reproductive health and rights (Mmari et al. 2014). Other studies of adolescent girls from urban slums have reported on their low levels of sexual and reproductive health knowledge (BoBhate et al. 2011; Masare et al. 2018; Kadạm et al. 2019) and low utilization of services for menstrual and other reproductive health problems (Muralidharan 2019).

Of the two studies which addressed female sex workers' sexual and reproductive health needs and service utilization (beyond HIV), one found that although female sex workers were the target group for interventions such as negotiating condom use with clients and treatment for HIV, they neither received antenatal HIV testing nor prevention of mother-to-child transmission (PMTCT) services (Becker et al. 2012). The other reported low use of barrier methods of contraception and emergency contraception and a high unmet need (74.3 per cent) for non-HIV sexual and reproductive health services (Lafort et al. 2017).

Thus, most of what one knows is that marginalized populations have poor access to health services and worse health outcomes than their better-off counterparts. The evidence provides just a few glimpses of the sexual and reproductive health experiences from the perspectives and lived experiences of women, adolescents, and young people from marginalized populations.

A rare study by Pawar (2022), who is from a nomadic tribe, provides an insider's view of how exclusion and marginalization at multiple levels impact the sexual and reproductive health of women from nomadic and denotified tribes (NT-DNT). The community faces deprivation of basic resources such as shelter, sanitation, identity documents, education, workplace safety, and transportation. Their struggle for survival, stigmatized status, and criminalization, as well as language barriers, make sexual and reproductive services inaccessible to them (Pawar 2022). Two studies from Odisha indicate a mismatch between the preferences of young married couples and women from tribal communities and the sexual and reproductive health programmes and services of the government (Palo et al. 2020; Contractor et al. 2018). Young tribal couples preferred to use withdrawal for spacing children; the government family planning services promoted the use of modern contraceptive methods such as the Intrauterine Device (IUD) and oral pills, which they distrusted, and female sterilization, which had low cultural acceptability (Palo et al. 2020). In the case of maternal health services, the government's conditional cash transfer programme for institutional delivery ignores the preference for home births for normal deliveries among tribal communities. Consequently, home births happen without skilled birth attendance. Institutional deliveries were not easily accessible even in the case of delivery complications because of the remote location of many tribal communities; those who opted for institutional deliveries found the environment alienating because of cultural and linguistic barriers (Contractor et al. 2018). Despite relative improvements in access to maternal health services because of the introduction of ASHAs as community-based workers, Dalit women from Bihar reported experiencing inequities and, at times, discrimination in maternal health services (Patel et al. 2018).

Access to safe abortion services is fraught with greater challenges than to maternal health services. A study from Tamil Nadu sought to examine the views of women from low income and socially marginalized groups on factors affecting access to safe abortion and choice of provider. These included cost, assurance of secrecy, promptness of service provision, absence of provider gatekeeping, and provider-imposed conditions, including compulsory acceptance of contraception for receiving abortion services (Sri & Ravindran 2012). Another study, also from Tamil Nadu, documents in detail the obstacle course that women from marginalized communities (among others) have to traverse to obtain abortion services. Providers were disrespectful of the women seeking abortion services and were often denied or delayed services. In government health facilities, abortion services were conditional on the acceptance of female sterilization (Sunil 2022).

In the context of India, urban slums are a clear example of social exclusion, characterized by poverty, inadequate housing, lack of access to basic services and social stigma. A study by Khanna et al. (2022) graphically illustrates how marginalization as migrant urban slum dwellers and patriarchal control over sexuality and reproduction compromises young women's sexual and reproductive rights. Poor health infrastructure and providers' indifferent attitudes erect additional barriers to young women's access to sexual and reproductive health care (Khanna et al. 2022).

Most studies about female sex workers' sexual and reproductive health in India have been from the vantage point of female sex workers as a high risk or 'key' population for HIV/AIDS. A recent (2022) study documents their voices on their need for and access to other sexual and reproductive health services such as contraception, abortion, pregnancy, and delivery care. Many female sex workers face difficulties in pregnancy detection. It may then be too late for an abortion or Prevention of mother to child transmission (PMTCT) services. The focus of health programmes is on HIV prevention to the exclusion of pregnancy prevention, and there is an unmet need for preventing unplanned pregnancies. Female sex workers also face barriers in accessing abortion services and sterilization because of health-care providers' insistence on spousal consent and the belief that these services are exclusively for legally married women (Shewal & Sahay 2022).

Thus, one has only fragments of evidence on sexual and reproductive health from the perspectives and experiences of women from marginalized population groups. This book adds to this sparse evidence base. It contains the stories of fifteen women of varying age groups from five different social and geographic locations, describing their lived experiences and voicing their health and other concerns from their distinctive vantage points, emerging from their economic exploitation, social exclusion, and cultural subordination.

The book demonstrates how economic, social, and interpersonal realities circumscribe and are intertwined with women's sexual and reproductive health experiences, including their interactions with the health-care system. In doing so, it highlights the centrality of the concept of 'sexual and reproductive justice' when addressing the sexual and reproductive health concerns of marginalized women.

Sexual and reproductive justice exists when

> all people have the power and the resources to make healthy decisions about their bodies, sexuality and reproduction. This means that every person has the right to
>
> (a) Choose to have or not have children
> (b) Choose the conditions under which to give birth or create a family
> (c) Care for their children with the necessary social support in a safe and healthy environment
> (d) Control their own body and self-expression, free from any form of sexual or reproductive oppression (City of New York 2024, web page)

Sexual and reproductive justice is not an opposing concept to sexual and reproductive rights. Rather, it is inclusive, highlighting the need to take into consideration the reality of women's existence to comprehend the forces shaping their sexual and reproductive health (Onwuachi-Saunders et al. 2019).

METHODOLOGY

The stories in this book were collected as part of a larger research project implemented during 2020-21 by CommonHealth—Coalition for Reproductive Health and Safe Abortion in India.[2]

The larger research project aimed to:

(a) Understand and document the sexual and reproductive health pathways which women from different marginalized groups have experienced during various reproductive life stages;

(b) Document any violations of sexual and reproductive rights at the household, community, and health system levels; and

(c) Examine the enablers and barriers in accessing care for sexual and reproductive health issues.

CommonHealth's worldview influenced what the study team set out to do and how they went about the larger study. CommonHealth understands health as socially determined and health inequalities as driven by political, economic, and social factors at multiple levels, from the global to the individual. Its focus is on structurally excluded population groups and they believe that social, economic, and political inequalities need to be eliminated for women and men to enjoy the highest attainable level of sexual and reproductive health and well-being—a perspective akin to the call for 'reproductive justice'.

The study was carried out by members of CommonHealth and consisted of four community-based organizations (CBOs) and one advocacy organization with community-based partners. These organizations conducted the studies in their respective field sites, where they have worked with local communities for several years and used their findings to inform their future activism and advocacy. One of the unique features of the study was the participatory processes of co-production of knowledge adopted throughout the study process. It was not a top down exercise but involved the study teams in all stages of the study, from defining the research questions to data analysis and report writing. For example, the tools for data collection were developed through a series of tool development workshops and data analysis and interpretation took place in workshops where CommonHealth members with research skills facilitated the process. Field data was collected by experienced field workers from the five organizations, using in-depth interviews with selected women over several sittings. Ethical clearance for the larger study was obtained from the

TABLE 1.1: DETAILS ON THE STUDY TEAMS, SITES AND POPULATIONS

Organisation Conducting the Study	*Study site*	*Study population*
The YP Foundation	North-east Delhi, Delhi Capital Territory	Young unmarried women from migrant Muslim and Hindu households in urban slums
SAHAJ	Vadodara, Gujarat	Young married and un-married women from migrant tribal households in urban slums
Rural Women's Social Education Centre	Tirukkazhukundrum taluk, Chengalpattu district, Tamil Nadu	Married rural women from Dalit households
Saheli Sangh	Pune, Maharashtra	Current and past female sex workers within and on the outskirts of Pune's red-light area
SAHAYOG	Odisha	Married women from Particularly Vulnerable Tribal Groups (PVTG) without Scheduled Tribe status on the outskirts of Bhubaneshwar

Source: CommonHealth, 2024.

Institutional Review Board of SAHAJ, and ethical norms were adhered to during the entire research process.

The stories included in this book are based on in-depth interviews conducted for the larger study. While each organization had carried out 5-10 in-depth interviews, it was decided to showcase the stories of a selected group of women from each site so that their distinct experiences are heard in their entirety, since the study report had synthesized the women's experiences. Fifteen stories, three from each site, were selected for inclusion in the book to represent a diversity of experiences. The selection of stories and decisions on how to transform the in-depth interview transcripts into coherent stories were made collectively in a CommonHealth workshop.

Once the stories were selected, the 'restory' method (Nasheeda et al. 2019) was used to transform the interviews into stories. The 'restorying' process consisted of immersing oneself in the transcript, plotting the chronology of events, and listening to the audio recording to fill in the gaps. The story was then rewritten in the third person, focusing on a key theme emerging from the story, with extracts from the interview to highlight critical issues (Nasheeda et al. 2019).

The stories were suitably anonymized. The authors have tried their best to remain faithful to each woman's story and respectful of her perspective. Each story was reviewed by a reviewer from CommonHealth who has been a part of the larger study and it went through several rounds of feedback and revision before being finalized.

The next five chapters contain the stories of these women, located against the backdrop of the states and districts where they reside. The seventh and final chapter draws together and reflects on the main themes emerging from these stories. The chapter ends with an emerging conceptual framework for ensuring reproductive justice and sexual health for the most marginalized, leaving no one behind.

NOTES

1. This is an unpublished scoping review covering studies on maternal health, safe abortion, adolescent, and young people's sexual and reproductive health and availability, access, affordability, and quality of sexual and reproductive health services.
2. CommonHealth is a network with members comprising individuals, community-based organizations, and other civil society organizations. It engages in evidence-based advocacy to promote access to sexual and reproductive health and safe abortion for all.

REFERENCES

Ali, B. & S. Chauhan (2020). 'Inequalities in the Utilisation of Maternal Health Care in Rural India: Evidences from National Family Health Survey III & IV'. *BMC Public Health, 20:* 369.

Ali, B., P. Debnath & T. Anwar (2021). 'Inequalities in Utilisation of Maternal Health Services in Urban India: Evidences from the National Family Health Survey-4'. *Clinical Epidemiology and Global Health, 10*: 100672.

Ansari, H. & R. Yeravdekar (2020). 'Respectful Maternity Care during Childbirth in India: A Systematic Review and Meta-analysis'. *Journal of Postgraduate Medicine, 66*(3): 133-40.

Aridoss, S., N. Jaganathasamy, A. Kumar, M. Natesan, R. Adhikary & E. Arumugam (2020). 'Socio-demographic Factors Associated with HIV Prevalence among Pregnant Women Attending Antenatal Clinics in Six Southern States of India: Evidence from the Latest Round of HIV Sentinel Surveillance'. *Indian Journal of Public Health, 64*(5): 26-31.

Aslam, M., T. Nawab, A. Ahmad, A.J. Abedi & S.A. Azmi (2022). 'Postpartum Depression and Its Clinico-social Correlates: A Community-based Study in Aligarh'. *Indian Journal of Public Health, 66*(4): 473-79.

Bango, M. & S. Ghosh (2022). 'Social and Regional Disparities in Utilization of Maternal and Child Healthcare Services in India: A Study of the Post-national Health Mission Period'. *Frontiers in Pediatrics*, 10: 895033.

Becker, M., S. Ramanaik, S. Halli, J.E. Blanchard, T. Raghavendra, P. Bhattacharjee, S. Moses, L. Avery & S. Mishra (2012). 'The Intersection between Sex Work and Reproductive Health in Northern Karnataka, India: Identifying Gaps and Opportunities in the Context of HIV Prevention'. *AIDS Research and Treatment*, 842576.

Bobhate, P.S. & S.R. Shrivastava (2011). 'A Cross-sectional Study of Knowledge and Practices about Reproductive Health among Female Adolescents in an Urban Slum of Mumbai'. *Journal of Family and Reproductive Health, 5*(4): 117-24.

Chintapalli, S. & I.J. Padmaja (2013). 'Seroprevalence of Toxoplasmosis in Antenatal Women with Bad Obstetric History'. *Tropical Parasitology 3*(1): 62-6.

City of New York. (2024). 'Sexual and Reproductive Justice' (web). https://www.nyc.gov/site/doh/health/health-topics/sexual-reproductive-justice-nyc.page

Contractor, S.Q., A. Das, J. Dasgupta & S. Van Belle (2018). 'Beyond the Template: The Needs of Tribal Women and Their Experiences with Maternity Services in Odisha, India'. *International Journal for Equity in Health*, *17*(1): 1-13.

Daniel, M., and F. Linder (2002). 'Marginal People'. In L. Breslow (ed.). *Encyclopedia of Public Health*, New York and Farmington Hills: Macmillan Reference USA.

David, J.K., R. Pant, R.R. Allam, V.P. Priya, S. Aridoss & E. Arumugam, (2020). 'The Relationship between Educational Attainment and HIV Prevalence among Pregnant Women attending Antenatal Clinics in Six States of India: Sentinel Surveillance from 2010 to 2017'. *Indian Journal of Public Health*, *64*(5): 5-21.

Fricker, Miranda. (2007). *Epistemic Injustice: Power and the Ethics of Knowing*. Oxford online edition. Oxford Academic. DOI: https://doi.org/10.1093/acprof:oso/9780198237907.001.0001.

George, M., A.R. Johnson & S. Thimmaiah (2022). 'Prevalence and Determinants of Antepartum Psychiatric Disorders: A Cross-sectional Study in 25 Villages of Sarjapur PHC area, Bangalore Urban District'. *Indian Journal of Social Psychiatry*, *38*(3): 264-9.

Jat, T.R., N. Ng & M.S. Sebastin (2011). 'Factors Affecting the Use of Maternal Health Services in Madhya Pradesh State of India: A Multilevel Analysis'. *International Journal for Equity in Health*: *10*(29): 1-11.

Jungari, S., B. Sharma & D. Wagh (2021). 'Beyond Maternal Mortality: A Systematic Review of Evidences on Mistreatment and Disrespect during Childbirth in Health Facilities in India'. *Trauma, Violence, and Abuse*, *22*(4): 739-51.

Kadam, D.D., U.S. Saurabha & S.C. Tiwari (2019). 'Health Needs of Adolescent Girls Living in an Urban Slum of a Metropolitan City: A Mixed Method Approach'. *Journal of Family Medicine and Prime Care*, *8*(8): 2661-6.

Kalra, H., T.D. Tran, L. Romero, P. Chandra & J. Fisher (2021). 'Prevalence and Determinants of Antenatal Common Mental Disorders among Women in India: A Systematic Review and Meta-analysis'. *Archives of Women's Mental Health*, *24*(1): 29-53.

Khanna, D., J.V. Singh, M. Agarwal & V. Kumar (2019). 'Bio-Social Characteristics as Determinants of Maternal Death: A Community-based Case-control Study'. *Indian Journal of Public Health Research and Development*, *10*(8): 23-7.

Khanna, R., M. Sheth, P. Talati, K. Damor & B. Chauhan (2022). 'Social and Economic Marginalisation and Sexual and Reproductive Health and Rights of Urban Poor Young Women: A Qualitative Study from Vadodara, Gujarat, India'. *Sexual and Reproductive Health Matters* [online], *29*(2): 2059898.

Kotdawala, K.P., M. Agrawal & P.A. Kotdawala (2022). 'Comparative Study of Bacterial Vaginosis in Preterm and Term Labor'. *Journal of South Asian Federation of Obstetrics and Gynaecology*, *14*(4): 361-4.

Kumar, A. & A. Singh (2016). 'Explaining the Gap in the Use of Maternal Healthcare Services between Social Groups in India'. *Journal of Public Health*, *38*(4): 771-81.

Kumar, G., T.S. Choudhary, A. Srivastava, R.P. Upadhyay, S. Taneja, R. Bahl, J. Martines, M.K. Bhan, N. Bhandari & S. Mazumder (2019). 'Utilisation, Equity and Determinants of Full Antenatal Care in India: Analysis from the National Family Health Survey-4'. *BMC Pregnancy and Childbirth*, *19*(1): 1-9.

Kumar, R. & A. Tewari (2018). 'Near-miss Obstetric Events and Its Clinico-social Correlates in a Secondary Referral unit of Burdwan District in West Bengal'. *Indian Journal of Public Health*, *62*(3): 235-8.

Lafort, Y., R. Greener, A. Roy, L. Greener, W. Ombidi, F. Lessitala, J. Skordis-Worrall, M. Beksinska, P. Gichangi, S. Reza-Paul, J.A. Smit, M. Chersich & M. Delva (2017). 'Sexual and Reproductive Health Services Utilization by Female Sex Workers is Context Specific: Results from a Cross-sectional Survey in India, Kenya, Mozambique and South Africa'. *Reproductive Health*, *14*(13): 1-10.

Masare, M.S., S.S. Divekar, S.M. Bhelkar & P.A. Hiwarkar (2018). 'Reforming the Perceptions about Reproductive Health amongst Adolescents in Urban Slums'. *International Journal of Community Medicine and Public Health*, *5*(6): 2458-63.

Mmari, K., R. Blum, F. Sonenstein, B. Marshall, H. Brahmbhatt, E. Venables, S. Delany-Moretlwe, C. Lou, E. Gao, R. Acharya, S. Jejeebhoy & A. Sangowawa (2014). 'Adolescents' Perceptions of Health from Disadvantaged Urban Communities: Findings from the WAVE Study. *Social Science and Medicine*, 104: 124-32. doi: 10.1016/j.socscimed.2013.12.012. Epub 2013 Dec 18. PMID: 24581070.

Mohanty, S.K., R.S. Mishra, S. Mishra & S. Sen (2020). 'Understanding Equity of Institutional Delivery in Public Health Centre by Level of Care in India: An Assessment using Benefit Incidence Analysis'. *International Journal for Equity in Health*, *19*(1): 1-20.

Muralidharan, A. (2019). 'Constrained Choices?: Menstrual Health and Hygiene Needs among Adolescents in Mumbai Slums'. *Indian Journal of Gender Studies*, *26*(1&2): 12-39.

Nasheeda, A., H.B. Abdullah, S.E. Krauss & N.B. Ahmed (2019). 'Transforming Transcripts into Stories: A Multimethod Approach to Narrative Analysis'. *International Journal of Qualitative Methods*, *18*: 1-9.

Onwuachi-Saunders, C., Q.P. Dang, J. Murray (2019). 'Reproductive Rights, Reproductive Justice: Redefining Challenges to Create Optimal Health for all Women'. *Journal of Healthcare, Science, and the Humanities*', *IX* (1): 19-31.

Palo, S.K., M. Samal, J. Behera & S. Pati (2020). 'Tribal Eligible Couple, and Care Providers' Perspective on Family Planning: A Qualitative Study in Keonjhar District, Odisha, India'. *Clinical Epidemiology and Global Health*, *8*(1): 60-5.

Panda, S.R., M. Jain & S. Jain (2018). 'Clinical Profile of Obstetric Patients Getting Admitted to ICU in a Tertiary Care Center having HDU Facility: A Retrospective Analysis'. *The Journal of Obstetrics and Gynecology of India*, *68*(6): 477-81.

Parida, S.P., A. Gajjala & P.P. Giri (2021). 'Empowering Adolescent Girls, is Sexual and Reproductive Health Education a Solution?' *Journal of Family Medicine and Primary Care*, *10*: 66-71.

Patel, P., M. Das & U. Das (2018). 'The Perceptions, Health-seeking Behaviours and Access of Scheduled Caste Women to Maternal Health Services in Bihar, India'. *Reproductive Health Matters*, *26*(54): 114-25.

Paul, S., S. Paul & K.S. James (2019). 'Universalisation versus targeting in Maternal and Child Health Care Provisioning: Evidence from India'. *SSM-Population Health*, *9*: 100502.

Pawar, D. (2022). 'From Criminalised Histories to Rightful Present– Nomadic Women Demand Equal Rights to Sexual and Reproductive Health: A Study in Maharashtra, India'. *Sexual and Reproductive Health Matters*, *29*(2): 2064051.

Raghavan, V., H.A. Khan, U. Seshu, S.P. Rai, J. Durairaj, G. Aarthi, C. Sangeetha, S. John & R. Thara (2021). 'Prevalence and Risk Factors of Perinatal Depression among Women in Rural Bihar: A

Community-based Cross-sectional Study'. *Asian Journal of Psychiatry*, *56*: 102552.

Rane, T.M., T.G. Mahanta, M. Baruah & S.D. Baruah (2019). 'Epidemiological Study of Maternal Death in Assam'. *Clinical Epidemiology and Global Health*, 7(4): 634-40.

Ravindran, S. & R. Gaitonde (2018). *Health Inequities in India: A Synthesis of Recent Evidence*. Singapore: Spinger.

Santhakumar, A., B. Ganesh, M. Malathi, J. Nagaraj, N. Manikandan, V.M. Padmapriya, B.K. Kirubakaran, C. Govindasamy, V. Ramachandran, R. Sridhar & P. Kumar (2020). 'Confined Vulnerability of HIV Infection among Pregnant Women Attending Antenatal Care Clinics in Karnataka, India: Analysis of Data from the HIV Sentinel Surveillance 2017'. *Clinical Epidemiology and Global Health*, *8*(4): 1127-33.

Sharma, H., S.K. Singh & S. Srivastava (2021). 'Spatial Heterogeneity and Major Correlates of Unmet Need of Family Planning among Young Married Women Aged 15-24 in India: An Exploratory Study'. *Sage Open*, *11*(2): 21582440211024615.

Sharma, P., Y. Marimuthu, S. Basu, N. Sharma, Y.M. Mala & B. Nagappa (2021). 'Intensified Case Finding for Screening Tuberculosis among Antenatal Women in Delhi, India; A Facility-based Prospective Observational Study'. *Clinical Epidemiology and Global Health*, *12*: 100816.

Shewale, S. & S. Sahay (2022). 'Barriers and Facilitators for Access and Utilization of Reproductive and Sexual Health Services among Female Sex Workers in Urban and Rural Maharashtra, India'. *Frontiers in Public Health*, *10*: 1030914.

Shivalli, S. & N. Gururaj (2015). 'Postnatal Depression among Rural Women in South India: Do Socio-demographic, Obstetric and Pregnancy Outcomes have a Role to Play?' *PloS One*, *10*(4): e0122079.

Singal, N., G. Setia, B.K. Taneja & K.K. Singal (2018). 'Factors Associated with Maternal Anaemia among Pregnant Women in Rural India'. *Bangladesh Journal of Medical Science*, *17*(4): 583-92.

Singh, I., A. Shukla, J.V. Thulaseedharan & G. Singh (2021). 'Contraception for Married Adolescents (15–19 years) in India: Insights from the National Family Health Survey-4 (NFHS-4)'. *Reproductive Health*, *18*(1): 1-10.

Singh, N., M.P. Singh, B.J. Wylie, M. Hussain, Y.A. Kojo, C. Shekhar, L. Sabin, M. Desai, V. Udhayakumar & D.H. Hamer (2012). 'Malaria Prevalence among Pregnant Women in Two Districts with Differing Endemicity in Chhattisgarh, India'. *Malaria Journal, 11:* 1-4.

Singh, P.K., R.K. Rai, M. Alagarajan & L. Singh (2012). 'Determinants of Maternity Care Services Utilization among Married Adolescents in Rural India'. *PloS one*, 7(2): e31666.

Singh, R., S.B. Neogi, A. Hazra, L. Irani, J. Ruducha, D. Ahmad, S. Kumar, N. Mann & D. Mavalankar (2019). 'Utilization of Maternal Health Services and Its Determinants: A Cross-sectional Study among Women in Rural Uttar Pradesh, India'. *Journal of Health, Population and Nutrition, 38*(13): 1-12.

Sri, B.S. & T.S. Ravindran (2012). 'Medical Abortion: Understanding Perspectives of Rural and Marginalized Women from Rural South India'. *International Journal of Gynecology & Obstetrics.* September, *118*: S33-9.

Sridharan, S., A. Dey, A. Seth, D. Chandurkar, K. Singh, K. Hay & R. Gibson (2017). 'Towards an Understanding of the Multilevel Factors Associated with Maternal Health Care Utilization in Uttar Pradesh, India'. *Global Health Action, 10*(1): 1287493.

Sunil, B. (2022). 'Running an Obstacle-course: A Qualitative Study of Women's Experiences with Abortion-seeking in Tamil Nadu, India'. *Sexual and Reproductive Health Matters, 29*(2): 1966218.

Swain, D., S.P. Parida, S.K. Jena, M. Das & H. Das (2020). 'Prevalence and Risk Factors of Obstetric Fistula: Implementation of a Need-based Preventive Action Plan in a South-eastern Rural Community of India'. *BMC Women's Health, 20*(40): 1-10.

Tanwar, R., S. Sarda, S. Agarwal & S. Dubey (2022). 'Prevalence of Sexually Transmitted Infection in Pregnancy at a Tertiary Care Center of Central India: An Observational Study'. *Journal of South Asian Federation of Obstetrics and Gynaecology, 14*(2): 128-31.

Tripathy, J.P. & S. Mishra (2017). 'Causes and Predictors of Neonatal, Post-neonatal and Maternal Deaths in India: Analysis of a Nationwide District-level Household Survey-4 (DLHS-4), 2012-13'. *Journal of Tropical Pediatrics, 63*(6): 431-39.

United Nations Population Fund (2019). *Sexual and Reproductive Health and Rights: An Essential Element of Universal Health Coverage.* https://www.unfpa.org/sites/default/files/pub-pdf/UF_SupplementAndUniversalAccess_30-online.pdf

Upadhyay, R.P., R. Chowdhury, A. Salehi, K. Sarkar, S.K. Singh, B. Sinha, A. Pawar, A.K. Rajalakshmi & A. Kumar (2017). 'Postpartum Depression in India: A Systematic Review and Meta-analysis'. *Bulletin of the World Health Organization*, *95*(10):706-171C.

Yadav, A.K., P.K. Jena, B. Sahni & D. Mukhopadhyay (2021). 'Comparative Study on Maternal Healthcare Services Utilisation in Selected Empowered Action Group States of India'. *Health and Social Care in the Community*, *29*(6): 1948-9.

Yadav, A.K., B. Sahni, P.K. Jena, D. Kumar & K. Bala (2020). 'Trends, Differentials, and Social Determinants of Maternal Health Care Services Utilization in Rural India: An Analysis from Pooled Data'. *Women's Health Reports*, *1*(1): 179-89.

CHAPTER 2

Stories of Young Women from North-east Delhi

SHRUTI ARORA, SOUVIK PYNE and ABHISHEK SEKARAN

Social norms and gender inequality pose huge barriers for young women's fulfilment of their sexual and reproductive rights (Plan International 2016). Discriminatory attitudes towards girls and young women mean that they are often denied the voice, agency, and autonomy to make their own decisions in relation to their sexual and reproductive health (SRH) (ibid.). Young women living in urban slums face intersectional barriers in realizing their sexual and reproductive health and rights (SRHR), not just due to their age and gender but also due to their poor economic situation. This chapter aims to explore how young women from the *basti*s of north-east Delhi negotiate social and gender norms to claim their sexual rights.

SEXUAL AND REPRODUCTIVE HEALTH IN NORTH-EAST DELHI

North-east Delhi has the highest population density in the country (36,155 persons per sq. km), and the highest concentration of informal low-income settlements or *basti*s among all the districts of the National Capital Territory (NCT) of Delhi (Census 2011). More than a third of the population are migrants from outside Delhi, living in congested kutcha or semi-pucca houses comprising barely a room or two (ibid.). Nearly 30 per cent of the population in this district are minorities, with Muslims being the predominant minority group (Hasan et al. 2008), living close to the poverty line (ibid.).[1]

In 2011, adolescents (aged 10-19 years) and young people (15-24 years) constituted 19 per cent and 20 per cent of the population of north-east Delhi, respectively; about 53 per cent of them were male and 47 per cent female (Census of India 2011). According to NFHS-4[2] (2015-16), a little over a tenth (12 per cent) of the young women aged 20-4 years were married before they were 18 and close to 3 per cent were already mothers or pregnant at the time of the survey. The proportion of young mothers in this area was higher than the average for the NCT of Delhi (IIPS & MOHFW 2015). The only study of young women living in *basti*s in north-east Delhi that the authors were able to identify is more than a decade old. This study of newly-married women indicated their poor overall and reproductive health status: more than three-fourths of them were anaemic and about a third reported menstrual complaints and reproductive tract infection (RTI) symptoms. Only about one-fifth said they used any form of contraception and a vast majority conceived within the first year of their marriage (Singh et al. 2010).

The district recorded 16 per cent non-skilled birth-attended home deliveries, 68 per cent normal institutional deliveries, and 15.3 per cent C-section deliveries (according to the Reproductive, Maternal, Newborn, Child Health and Adolescent Health (RMNCHA) performance conducted under the Delhi Health Mission in 2013-14). The district has 25 Delhi government primary urban health centres, one district hospital, one facility operated under the Central Government Health Scheme, six maternal and child welfare centres operated under the Municipal Corporation of Delhi, one NGO-led health facility, and 14 private health facilities. However, the availability of infrastructure and services at these centres is unclear (District performance 2013-14).

ADOLESCENT HEALTH PROGRAMMES IN THE REGION

In 2014, the Delhi government announced that north-east Delhi was a high-priority district under the Rashtriya Kishor

Swasthya Karyakram (RKSK). It launched DISHA clinics under RKSK guidelines and adolescent-friendly health clinics (AFHCs) at the primary, secondary, and tertiary levels, the objective being to improve nutrition and sexual and reproductive health, enhance mental health, prevent injuries, violence and, substance abuse, and address conditions for non-communicable diseases (NCDs). However, alarmingly, there is very little awareness about the existence of the DISHA clinics and AFHCs amongst adolescents (Santhya et al. 2014; Human Rights Law Network (HRLN) 2018). Only about 5 per cent of young men and 8 per cent of young women were aware of the AFHCs in a 5-10 km radius of their homes (Santhya et al. 2014). Some of the key challenges that young people reported in accessing services are the conservative and patriarchal attitudes and beliefs of health-care providers on adolescent sexuality, homosexuality, and pre-marital sex; the lack of privacy and confidentiality at the clinics; non-availability of same-gender service providers; poor Water, Sanitation and Hygiene (WASH) facilities; lack of Information, Education and Communication (IEC) materials; and, where available, the focus on family planning with no information on menstrual health, nutrition, premarital safe sex, abortion, etc. (The YP Foundation 2019). The study also found that apart from the AFHC component of the RKSK programme, none of its other community outreach components had been rolled out by the government. It is important to note that while SRH finds a focus in the programme, the national Protection of Children from Sexual Offences (POCSO) Act criminalizes consensual sexual activity before the age of 18 and mandates service providers to report such cases to the police. This contradiction in policies, therefore, undermines adolescents' decision-making capacities and their right to access to SRH services confidentially.

While there are several NGOs working in the district, the two key interventions involving young women are being led by the grassroots organizations, Action India and Sewa. Action India works on violence against women and gender issues within the slum communities of north-east Delhi, with menstrual health being a strong component of their work. Between 2018 and 2021, Action India and The YP Foundation worked on a programme to assess the youth friendliness of SRH services and to improve young people's knowledge and access to SRH. It used a youth-led model where young people themselves audited the AFHCs in their areas. Action India also ran an education centre for girls who were school drop-outs in collaboration with Nirantar at the time of data collection. Sewa runs computer centres for young women from the community at subsidised rates. Between 2017 and 2019, Sewa and The YP Foundation collaborated to form collectives of young women to build their leadership skills so that they could advocate with community leaders and other stakeholders for their rights.

Given this context, the three stories presented here offer different insights into the lives of young women from this district. The stories highlight the pathways taken by young women in the fulfilment of sexual (and reproductive) rights and their aspirations, negotiations, and resistance to pervasive gender and sexual norms.

'IF I INTRODUCE MY MOTHER AND BOYFRIEND TO EACH OTHER, I WILL ACTUALLY HAVE TO MARRY HIM': FALGUNI'S STORY

Falguni is 19 years old, studying in Class 11 in a government school. She is from a Muslim, Pathan (general) caste family. Unlike most households in Nand Nagri, she lives with her mother in a single-parent home.

Falguni and her mother had moved to Delhi from a village near Kanpur in Uttar Pradesh to live with her *nani* (maternal grandmother) after her mother's divorce. They shared a house with her *nani*, *khaala* (maternal aunt), *mamu* (maternal uncle), and his four daughters. She spent most of her childhood with her *nani* and *mamu* and felt very connected to them. As she grew older, she began experiencing the changing dynamics of the family. Her *nani* and *khaala*, suspecting she had a boyfriend, would watch her and follow her to her tuition centre to 'prove she had a boyfriend'. When they could find no evidence, they simply asserted she had a boyfriend, which triggered a fight between her mother and her *nani;* her mother told her *nani* to stop restricting Falguni's mobility and the way she dressed. When things escalated a year ago, her mother decided to move to a one-room rented house with a toilet and a kitchen but no bathroom.

Falguni is very close to her mother, who is an outlier in their society, having fought against gender norms and leaving two abusive marriages before moving to Delhi. While Falguni does not remember witnessing domestic violence in her mother's marriages, she recalls her *mamu* hitting her and her mother when they lived with her *nani*. She is hurt by what her *nani* and *khaala* did, and she and her mother are no longer in contact with her *nani*, *khaala*, and *mamu* now. She only meets her two cousins as they study in the same school.

She is able to wear jeans and T-shirt now; her *nani* would insist she wore only *salvar kameez*. While she would hear her *nani* tell her male cousins (her *khaala*'s sons) to 'find girls of your choice to marry', this was something Falguni had never been told. 'In fact, she only suspects and accuses me of having a boyfriend', she says. One could imagine that Falguni would enjoy the freedom of living in a small family set up now, but she says,

> My mother goes to work and I am alone at home. It is better to live in a joint family set-up with cousins. I miss them and I don't like living alone.

Her mother earns around Rs. 7,000 a month working in a stationery factory a few km from their home. Falguni has a younger brother who is a drug addict; his friends, other young men in the community, are also addicts. He has been missing for six months and they have not been able to find him. Falguni likes going to school. Her best friend there is a Hindu girl with whom she shares all her secrets. She aspires to be an office manager or a police officer. The television shows she has seen (such as *Diya aur Baati* and *Afsar Bitiya* with stories centred around young female protagonists), have inspired and influenced her.

She was 15-16 at the onset of menarche; she was prepared for it by the sessions on menstruation in school. When she first got her period, she told a friend who helped her with a sanitary napkin and she had no problem telling her mother about her period. Initially she had severe period pains, which have reduced over the years but are still quite severe. She has not visited a doctor for the pain, saying,

> As long as I am around people, I do not feel the pain but it worsens when I am sitting alone.

On various occasions, she and her mother have discussed their menstruation experiences. She is comfortable with her other bodily changes, such as the development of breasts, as she expects that her body will eventually look like other women's bodies.

Falguni recalled that it took a lot of negotiation with her *nani* before she was allowed to go to the NGO centre to attend computer classes and gender sessions. There she learnt about menstruation, contraception usage, safe abortion and intimate partner violence, from a women's rights perspective. Since she has never had a sexual relationship, she has not used contraception. She is not enthusiastic about negotiating contraception use with her future partner, because the thought of sex disgusts her. She wonders aloud how women can enjoy something like sex, reasoning that 'maybe with time, they get used to it'.

She remembers the first time she felt attracted to a boy. He lives in her community and they played together, but when her bodily changes started becoming visible, her family stopped her from playing with boys. The boy tries to contact her, but she doesn't take his calls as she had heard that his intentions were to brag to his peers that they were having an affair.

Like many schoolgirls in Nand Nagri, Falguni goes for tuition classes. She broke up with her boyfriend of two years (who she met in her tuition classes) because he wanted to have sex. She was heartbroken that her boyfriend did not want to continue their relationship without expecting sex.

Having sex with him would have meant breaking her mother's trust. She does not regret prioritizing her mother's values in the conflict between what her boyfriend wanted and what her mother expected. She wonders if there are boys for whom feelings and emotions are equally or more important than sex.

Falguni has a smartphone; ever since her breakup she has been talking to other boys on Facebook and WhatsApp. She befriended one boy through Facebook and met another in a hospital where they exchanged phone numbers to continue talking through WhatsApp. She feels that boys on Facebook cannot be trusted, but as she is single now, she uses these apps for 'time-pass', implying casual relationships.

Falguni's mother knew about her earlier boyfriend. She had not opposed their relationship and in fact, had wanted to meet him; Falguni had felt some pressure from her mother to marry him. She noted that while her mother was progressive in allowing her to enter into a relationship, she had also counselled her to 'not do anything that would let her down, bring shame or dishonour . . . or give an opportunity for her *nani* to point a finger at them', indirectly suggesting that she should not have sex, get pregnant, or run away with someone. Falguni feels that she cannot take advantage of the liberty her mother has given her. She has a strong inclination to retain/uphold her mother's trust. She says,

> There is no forgiving for pre-marital sex in our religion. Second, if people find out, *ammi-abbu* lose their face in the eyes of society. It is better to not do it instead of regretting it later.

The idea of marriage does not interest Falguni and she wants to continue living with her mother. When asked if she could live her life without being married (as she states) and have only 'time-pass boyfriends' (who she meets online), she knew the answer. Her mother may not have a problem if she does not marry, but she will not allow her to date boys casually. Neither her mother nor other members of her family would accept her dating without the intention of marriage. She laughingly says, 'if I introduce my mother and the guy to each other, I will actually have to marry him'.

MARRIAGE AS THE WAY OUT OF DIRE POVERTY AND PARENTAL CONTROL? PINKY'S STORY

Pinky is 21 years old and lives in Nand Nagri. She belongs to a 'general caste' Hindu family. She is the second daughter in a family of four daughters and two younger sons. It has not been easy for her to grow up in a family of four daughters.

Her father is a street vendor. They live with her paternal uncles and her parents and six siblings occupy only one room in the house. There are frequent fights with her cousins due to the cramped space and she feels suffocated. There is no toilet in the house; the community toilets they have to use do not receive a regular supply of water, and are not opened or cleaned regularly. When she wants to use the toilet, either her mother or her sister has to go with her, especially in the evening and at night.

She recalls the animosity her mother faced as her parents could not have children for the first five years of their marriage. When they first had three daughters, her mother continued to face violence due to the son preference norms in their society. She elaborates,

> My father's family called her *baanjh* (infertile). After five years of their marriage when my elder sister was born, they separated her and my mother. They did not give them anything to eat. Then they had three daughters. . . . My father started drinking more and more. He started beating up and shouting at my mother after drinking.

Her father is an alcoholic and abuses her mother even now. The only way out of the dire circle of violence and poverty she can see for her parents is to take their share of the joint property and buy another house. However, with three unmarried daughters, including herself, the money they receive will not cover the expense of purchasing a new house as well as getting them married. She feels extremely stressed:

All the extended family members are telling my father to buy a new house this year with the money he will get by selling the joint family house. And then they can marry me off next year. How will they manage money for both? He cannot spend all the money on my marriage either; my brothers should also not have a problem in the future if our father does not make a house for them. This is my biggest tension. I have a headache thinking about all this. I often take medicine for the headache.

Pinky was trained in a beauty parlour and in tailoring after completing her Class X, but she is not allowed to practise either professionally. She missed the deadline for admission to Class XI as the family had to go to the village because her father's brother passed away. She missed the application for admission the next year too as her father's second brother passed away. After that her father did not allow her to go to school. Pinky's sister too was not allowed to continue her schooling when she failed in Class IX.

Despite desperate and difficult economic conditions, her father does not allow her to work in a beauty parlour, since it is not a tradition in their family. Pinky elaborates,

I did the parlour course but there was no space to open a parlour. Then I learnt stitching but did not get space to do that professionally either. I have killed my heart's desires. The entire issue is about space, there is no space where I can practise. . . . They do not allow me to go and work outside. I told my mother that I found a parlour to work in, it is very close to our house. But my father did not allow me to go. . . . He only listens to his family and traditions. He said that I would be gone from home for eight hours. If it is 2-3 hours of work, they were fine. I also have a lot of students who want to learn stitching, but there is no space at home for me to do that.

Pinky, along with her mother and younger sister, do home based stitching and making plastic bags (*lifafa*s). She has a small sewing machine and would like to buy a bigger one. Above all, she aspires to learn English and computers. There is a computer centre close by, run by an NGO, but she cannot afford the monthly fee of Rs. 400. Even though she desperately wants to move out of the house they live in, she wants to learn computers and English before they move.

Pinky was 12 at the onset of menarche and did not know about it in advance. Her mother and elder sister explained it is a monthly occurrence and showed her how to use sanitary pads. She sometimes uses a cloth when she does not have a sanitary pad, but that is very rare. Given their cramped living space, she has no privacy to change her sanitary pads. She also experiences very severe menstrual pains, which confine her to bed, sometimes for three days. She has not consulted a doctor for this, but her mother gives her pain-killers.

When she started menstruating, her parents told her that as she had 'become mature', she should stop going out alone in the evenings and not wear pants or *pyjama*s. She wishes she could go back to wearing pants and remembers her childhood:

> I was a healthy child. I had a boy's haircut and dressed in pant shirt. Since there were no boys in the family, my father treated me like a boy.

Being treated as a boy made her feel special in the family. Those are her most pleasant memories and she reminisces about the love, care, and freedom childhood had symbolized.

She was attracted to a Muslim boy who lives in their neighbourhood. They would kiss; he wanted to have sexual intercourse, but she refused initially and avoided meeting him in secluded places. Eventually they began a relationship and she had her first sexual experience with him. When they had been together for a year, they were seen together by neighbours and her younger sister, who told her parents. Pinky was severely reprimanded:

> My mother told me, your honour is in your own hands. All of that has to happen (meaning sex). You will get married, that thing will also happen. I promised that day I would not repeat it. I still see that boy but I don't want to do anything now.

The boy wanted to marry her, but her parents would not have agreed as he is Muslim. Pinky was also unsure about marrying him, because she felt controlled by him and he seemed to stalk her constantly when she went out. She broke up with him after her parents learnt about their relationship.

Pinky met a suitor at her sister's wedding. He is her *bua*'s (paternal aunt's) son and grew up in a village, but now works as a driver in the city. Pinky likes him and her family also approves of their relationship. The arranged-cum-love marriage situation means that she does not have to hide things from her parents, as in her previous relationship. She feels a certain desperation to get married as it will be an escape from the tense environment of her home. She would like to continue to live in the city after her marriage and not move to the *sasural* (husband's village). She would like him to stop being a non-vegetarian after their marriage, but he says he will teach her to be a non-vegetarian. She fears that her family's poor living conditions may put her in a position where she may not be able to negotiate.

'WHAT KIND OF GIRL AM I WHO GOT PREGNANT BEFORE MARRIAGE?' RUKMINI'S STORY

Rukmini is 19 years old; for the past few months she has been living in the premises of an NGO office where she has a full-time job. She had not planned on joining the NGO or on working on women's rights. She used to live with her parents in Seemapuri, giving tuitions to children. Her life took a drastic turn when she found out she was pregnant. She had to escape from home before the news of an unmarried girl's pregnancy spread in her family and community. She gave birth to her baby in a private hospital and gave him up for adoption. Her premarital pregnancy exposed her to a societal harshness that not many girls of her age would know about.

Like many other young women in her community, her family had migrated to Delhi from Bihar. They are from a Hindu general caste, and her father works in a car manufacturing company and her mother in a tailor's shop. Her parents own a one-room house in the slums of Seemapuri, where they live with Rukmini and her two brothers. Rukmini studied in a government school and although she was doing well in her studies, she failed her Class XII board exams. Ashamed about going back to school, she did not reappear for her exams and discontinued her studies.

She has faced community surveillance from neighbours. It angered her when they would tattle to her mother if they saw her and other young women in the park, as her mother started placing restrictions on her, constantly telling her not to talk to boys.

She was 12 at the onset of menarche, still living in the village in Bihar. Nobody had explained to her what menstrual periods were. It was only much later when she started visiting the NGO centre that she learnt why menstruation happens and the myths around it. She had not known that sex could lead to pregnancy.

Rukmini had her first relationship when she was 16 with a boy who lived in the same neighbourhood. He was two years older, and worked in a chicken shop. He was a Bengali but she did not know his caste. She liked talking to him as she was lonely and had no one to share her feelings with. When her father and brother found out about the relationship, they did not approve, and reprimanded her saying that the boy was from a lower class, so she should break her off contacts with him.

Rukmini felt that she did not have an equal say in her relationship with the boy, who pressured her twice into having unprotected sex. She stressed that he could have used protection:

> He asked to me to have sex after we had been together for two years. . . . I did not want to, but I couldn't say yes nor no. At the time of sex, I really did not know that a pregnancy could happen. I did not think that if we had sex, he should use protection. I thought he would take care of everything.

She discovered she was expecting quite late in her pregnancy:

> I think we had sex in the month of December. I did not realize that I was pregnant. I just continued with my everyday schedule, teaching tuitions.

My boyfriend and I started quarrelling a lot during this time, so I stopped talking to him. Sometime in April, my *nani* came to Delhi, and I returned to the village with her. I did not pay attention when I skipped my period. My bump started showing when I was still in the village . . . but I would tell people that I had a swelling in my stomach. . . . They believed me, nobody ever doubted me because to them I was a very good girl. When I came back to Delhi that is when I decided to do something.

When she started feeling the foetus moving in her womb, she decided to tell a friend who got her some medical abortion pills. When the friend looked at her pregnancy though, she suggested not taking the pills but visiting the doctor as the pregnancy had become quite visible by then. The friend took her to a gynaecologist who refused to terminate the pregnancy as she was already 34 weeks pregnant. After her visit to the doctor, Rukmini feared people's reactions:

What would everybody say, what kind of a girl I am who got pregnant before marriage? I did not know how to tell people, what to say.

When Rukmini told her boyfriend about the pregnancy, he suggested eloping and getting married, but she did not want to do that. She decided instead to speak to a women's rights activist she knew, who worked in her community. The activist promised to help her through her NGO, but by then Rukmini's neighbour had noticed her bump and remarked to her brother that it looked as if she had been eating for two. That night Rukmini's mother and brother pestered her with questions, but she refused to speak with them; her father was out at work. She decided to ask her activist friend to help her leave home the next morning.

The activist came the next morning to ask her father for permission to take her for a residential workshop. This was not easy, but Rukmini managed to get out. The NGO supported her in getting her tests done. Her test reports were normal, but she had to hide her bump for another month. With her informed consent, the NGO arranged for her stay, medical expenses, and delivery and for the adoption of her baby. She lived at the home of the head of the NGO until her delivery.

She had a normal delivery, about a month after living away from home. She was treated very respectfully at the hospital because the NGO was involved. As she was over 18, she could sign the adoption papers without needing permission from a guardian. The NGO invited her father to the NGO office and informed him about Rukmini's pregnancy and delivery. He was extremely angry, saying he would have nothing to do with his daughter. Going back to live with her parents was not an option because of the scandal she had caused.

Her premarital pregnancy changed Rukmini's life and her perception of herself in many ways. She had been viewed as a sincere, good girl by her neighbours, teachers, and other community members. 'My life turned upside down when my own parents ostracised me', she says, when describing the harrowing experience of leaving her home and the community.

Since then, Rukmini has been focusing on her own learning and growth in an attempt to become financially independent. She earns Rs. 5,000 to 6,000 per month, has control over her own income and makes her own decisions on how to spend her money. She has occasionally gone home to visit her parents, but they have still not forgiven her. She stopped giving tuitions, something she had enjoyed quite a lot, and wonders if she will ever be able to do that again. She also wonders if she will find a partner who will be able to accept her after this life event. She feels dejected and has no interest in forming a romantic relationship or getting married in the near future. But she is certain she wants to continue working with the NGO to help build confidence in other young women.

CONCLUSIONS FROM THESE WOMEN'S STORIES

While one knows enough about young married women's challenges in accessing reproductive health and rights, very little is known about young unmarried women's sexual experiences related to their health and rights. Stigma and shame around these issues add layers of barriers even for researchers to research these topics. The focus of this chapter has been on understanding marginalized young unmarried women's lived experiences of gender and sexuality.

These stories highlight the experiences of young women exploring their sexuality. The young women whose stories were shared in this chapter, live in a culture where patriarchal control over women's bodies and sexuality is the norm and there is a serious price to pay for digressions from these gendered sexual norms. Adhering to the norms usually means getting rewards and privileges in the form of love, respect, independence, and money. This patriarchal model of reward for adhering and punishment for digression, is a huge barrier to independent decision making, especially for women, and particularly when it comes to if, when, and who they marry and in the actualization of their other sexual rights.

These three case stories also show that young women's desires and expectations of gender equal intimate relations with men is not easily fulfilled. They have little information about their bodies and sexuality, conception, and contraception. All they know is that interacting with boys could bring dishonour to their families. Their boyfriends' insistence on having sex when they know that women bear the brunt of losing 'family honour' and their lack of responsibility for contraception, exposes the gendered nature of sexual relations, desires, and sexuality. Rukmini's story points compellingly to male coercion in sex; but whereas young men are socially protected for initiating premarital sex, young women are made to pay the price.

Falguni's exploration of her sexuality by going on dates with boys, facilitated by Facebook chats, breaks stereotypical perceptions of Muslim women's sexual freedom. Her mother is an outlier in society: her openness to a love marriage suggests that the norms around finding a groom may be slowly changing. But then, 'respectable girls' must marry their boyfriends. There is little scope for a girl to object to marriage if news of her having a boyfriend reaches the family. This indicates that while practices such as love marriages may be becoming more acceptable among the younger generation, it does not mean that young women enjoy sexual rights.

Love marriages are acceptable, if at all, only within the same caste and religion. Pinky's story illustrates the community's continued restriction of interreligious romantic and sexual relationships and that maintaining woman's chastity and consummation of their relationship post-marriage is still of importance for family honour.

As seen in Rukmini's story, premarital pregnancy has severe consequences in the form of the withdrawal of family and community support that women depend on in the Indian context. Marriage becomes a precondition for women to access SRH services. The lack of knowledge, judgemental attitude of family members, and fear of being labelled a 'bad woman' result in a delay in women seeking a safe abortion. Additionally, the absence of any state sponsored protection and support systems for women who may have a premarital pregnancy or who may challenge other gender and sexual norms, is a form of state apathy and a denial of female sexual rights.

For young women living in poor economic conditions, the intersectionality of gender, age, and economic status defines how they experience sexual and reproductive health. This is evident from Pinky's narrative describing the cramped housing and hygiene conditions of the community toilets, her painful menstruation/poor menstrual health, the burden of unpaid domestic labour, and her vulnerability to domestic violence within the household. It is not only parental control she experiences, but also the lack of space within her home which restricts her livelihood opportunities and keeps her home-bound and dependent. For her, an arranged marriage appears to be the only route to escape the suffocating circumstances of her life, even if it is a risky one. While the economic situations of Rukmini and Falguni are not so dire, their positions as young women in low-income households within a patriarchal social setting restrict the investment their families are willing to make in them, limiting their life opportunities, and constraining their ability to exercise their sexual rights.

NGOs often face a severe backlash and gatekeeping from parents of young women, especially when it comes to imparting information about sex and sexuality before marriage. They play a critical role as they are the only formal form of support available for women like Rukmini, when all other social or formal support systems are inaccessible. At the same time, it also needs to be acknowledged that not all women are able to negotiate accessing NGO centres. Young women's lives and needs are heterogeneous: for young women from very poor backgrounds, the burden of domestic work and time constraints add an extra barrier to their learning about sexuality; for young Muslim women, the preconceived notions of Islam being against premarital sex adds a layer of complexity in developing a rights-based and pleasure-based attitude towards their own sexuality.

The silver lining in this gloomy scenario is the resilience of the young women, despite how poverty and patriarchy play out in their lives. They have high aspirations about many things: going back to learning and studying computers or English, finding a job, or becoming financially independent.

NOTES

1. The sexual and reproductive health experiences of the young women in this population needs to be viewed against the backdrop of insecurity and vulnerability owing to communal tensions, predominantly affecting the Muslim households. North-east Delhi was the centre of targeted violence on 24-26 February 2020, after data collection for the study.
2. These are the latest available figures. NFHS-5 data on age at first marriage and teenage pregnancy are not available by district.

REFERENCES

Government of India (2011). Census 2011. *District Census Handbook: NCT of Delhi.* New Delhi: Directorate of Census Operations. Available at: https://censusindia.gov.in/nada/index.php/catalog/913

Government of India (web portal) (2023). District performance (2013-14), North East Delhi, RMNCHA. Health Management Information System, Government of India. Available at: https://dshm.delhi.gov.in/(S(q1brmvk2bjup4rdqhei41jjg))/pdf/md_HMIS_16_indiDesh/North%20East%20 District_16_dashboard_ind_2013-14.pdf

Hasan, M., A. Razzack, T. Fazal, K. Kaur & S. Saeed (2008). *Baseline Survey of North-east District, NCT Delhi.* New Delhi: Ministry of Minority Affairs, Government of India.

Human Rights Law Network (HRLN). (2018). *RKSK's DISHA clinics for adolescents in Delhi.* Reproductive Rights Initiative. Available at: http://reproductiverights.hrln.org/wp-content/uploads/2018/09/AFHC-Fact-Finding-Mission-Report-Edit-13092018.pdf

Plan International. (2016). *Sexual and Reproductive Health and Rights.* Available at: https://plan-international.org/uploads/2021/12/srhr_position_paper_-io-eng-jun17-final.pdf

Santhya, K.G., S. Jejeebhoy, R. Prakash & S.K. Singh (2014). *Accessing Adolescent Friendly Health Clinics in India: The Perspectives of Adolescents and Youth.* New Delhi: Population Council.

Singh, S., S. Chaturvedi, A.T. Kannan & A. Kumar (2010). 'Reproductive Health of Newly Married Women Residing in a Resettlement Colony of Delhi: A Longitudinal Study'. *Indian Journal of Public Health:* 30-2.

The YP Foundation. (2019). *Youth-led Audits for Strengthening Adolescent and Youth-friendly Health Services.* New Delhi: The YP Foundation.

CHAPTER 3

Young Urban Adivasi Women from Vadodara, Gujarat

MANUSHI SHETH, ANAGHA PRADHAN and RENU KHANNA

AN OVERVIEW OF ADOLESCENTS' AND YOUNG WOMEN'S SRHR IN GUJARAT

Gujarat is recognized as an economically prosperous and infrastructurally developed state, and as one of the well-governed states in western India. However, it lags behind similar states in its social indicators, including those related to gender equality. Deep-rooted cultural and social practices like early and forced marriages, female youth illiteracy and caste discrimination are more evident in Gujarat than in other states and add to the vulnerability of its young population (Ganeshan 2020).

Gujarat's female sex ratio at birth has been deteriorating.[1] Around 22 per cent of women aged 20-24 are married before the age of 18 and less than half the urban girls (47.9 per cent) make it to secondary school and complete ten years of schooling (NFHS-5).[2]

Its health system is one of the better ones in the country: the most recent Sustainable Development Goals (SDG) India Index has assigned the state the top rank on SDG-3 (*Ensure Health and Well Being*) United Nations Development Programme (UNDP & NITI Aayog 2021). Despite this, its health indicators are found to be wanting. High levels of malnutrition and anaemia have been long-standing problems: 65 per cent of women aged 15 to 49 are anaemic (NFHS-5), and anaemia has worsened in the last five years. Only around 54 per cent of married women use modern methods of contraception. Access to safe abortions and contraceptives remain services with little or no scope for informed choice for the young population. Awareness about the physiology of menstruation, symptoms of and access to health care for reproductive tract infections (RTIs), conception, and contraception is low among adolescent girls (aged 10-15 years) across the state. The state especially fails to cater to the needs of vulnerable women and girls in remote areas and among the urban poor. For example, two important adolescent-focused health programmes, SABLA[3] and the Rashtriya Kishore Swasthya Karyakram (RKSK)[4] are not available in urban areas, and since its inception, RKSK has been a pilot programme in only ten districts out of 33 in the state.

Vadodara is the third-largest city in Gujarat. Surrounded by several industrial areas, it attracts migrants from neighbouring districts and states, who now comprise over one-third of the city's population. They are among the most marginalized groups in the slum areas, and account for about 5 per cent of the city's total population (Vadodara City Population 2023). Public health-care services in Vadodara city are primarily provided through two government tertiary (medical college) hospitals, 19 urban health centres, and 15 full- and part-time dispensaries. While the urban health network of the Vadodara Municipal Corporation is reasonably good, it does not serve particularly the sexual and reproductive health (SRH) needs of women and girls and most of them rely on commercial private health services or the tertiary medical college hospital. Neither the RKSK nor SABLA is implemented in urban Vadodara.[5] Currently, only the Mamta Taruni Abhiyan,[6] limited to girls aged between 10 and 19 years, operates in the low-income neighbourhoods of the city. The beneficiaries are a selected group of 20 girls enrolled in the *anganwadi* records.

There are three cadres of health workers in the system. The *anganwadi* worker (AWW) is supposed to disseminate SRH information, but this usually covers only two topics, menstruation and nutrition. Peer educators selected by the AWW are only supposed to mobilise adolescents to utilize the services, they do not have any role as educators or guides.

The *anganwadi*s also provide 'take-home rations' or supplementary nutrition to the 20 enrolled girls. ASHAs, the second cadre of frontline workers, focus mainly on certain target-oriented tasks for married women (including adolescents and young women) related to antenatal and post-natal care and contraception. Although the ASHA is supposed to stock sanitary pads that the girls can buy at subsidized rates, they often have no stock. The third cadre, ANMs (Auxiliary Nurse Midwives), are tasked with conducting sessions with adolescent girls on menstrual health problems, nutrition, and the care of children under five. The sessions take place during the monthly Mamta Divas (Maternity Day), and the ANMs have to manage these within their already packed schedule of antenatal check ups and vaccination for children.

Adolescent SRH clinics are conducted at the Urban Primary Health Centres (UPHCs) and ward-level Community Health Centres on Mondays, 3-5 p.m. for girls and Tuesdays, 3-5 p.m. for boys. The UPHCs have either a male or a female doctor, but not both, so the boys' clinics will not necessarily have a male doctor; boys often feel embarrassed about open discussions with a female doctor. Adolescent Reproductive and Sexual Health (ARSH) services typically consist of dispensing medicines and giving information or dosage, but not providing information or counselling; for their SRH needs, adolescents prefer going to private practitioners, most of whom have non-allopathic degrees.

Basic health and sexuality education is missing from the school curriculum; biology topics in textbooks (reproductive organs, menstruation, conception, and contraception) contain technical language, inappropriate terms, and inadequate explanations. For example, RTIs/STIs find their place in the chapter on the excretory system (Gujarat state curriculum). Teachers skip these topics in class, and questions on these are designated as choice questions in exams, conveying the point that they are unimportant.

Clearly, the urban poor, specifically young girls and women in Vadodara, are vulnerable in terms of not having their needs addressed. There is also limited published research on the quality of SRH health services provided through the public health system in urban Vadodara. The few existing studies on health programmes for adolescent girls and young women have focused only on services to pregnant women and lactating mothers. However, the studies conducted in urban Vadodara echoed the SAHAJ team's observations about the inadequacies of health-care delivery to adolescent girls and young women. An observational study of the Mamta Divas in urban Vadodara noted the absence of staff and equipment, and the unsatisfactory levels of knowledge and skills among the staff examining pregnant women (Mehta et al. 2016). This study did not explore the quality of services provided to adolescent girls. Another large study (Kotecha & Karkar 2009) noted that over half the urban adolescent schoolgirls were anaemic despite availing Weekly Iron Folic Acid Supplementation (WIFS); and yet another study (Nambiar et al. 2012) found that only half the registered adolescents availed of midday meals. These findings hint at systemic problems within the health-care delivery system, which could also be applicable to the SRH care services provided through government-implemented programmes.

This chapter is based on action research carried out with young women from urban marginalized communities by the Society for Health Alternatives (SAHAJ), a Vadodara-based NGO. SAHAJ has over three decades of experience, working with underprivileged communities from 23 slums/*basti*s, especially women and adolescents, empowering them to bring positive changes in their lives.

The populations in the *basti*s where SAHAJ works, consist mainly of socially and economically vulnerable groups—Scheduled Castes (SCs), Other Backward Castes (OBCs) and Scheduled Tribes (STs), migrants from neighbouring states (such as Maharashtra and Madhya Pradesh) and the neighbouring tribal districts of Dahod, Panchmahal and Mahisagar, daily wage labourers, and unskilled workers. Many of these *basti*s are not 'recognized' by the city administration, meaning they have no 'official' electricity, water or sewage connections. They are densely populated and overcrowded, and prone to floods. In terms of health services, these residents are among the most needy and underserved populations.

Against this background, a study titled 'Reproductive health histories of young women of marginalized communities of Vadodara' was undertaken by SAHAJ with support from CommonHealth—Coalition of Reproductive Health and Safe Abortion (CH). The following three stories portray the SRH experiences of poor urban young women and the barriers and enablers to their enjoyment of sexual and reproductive rights.

A LIFE WITHOUT CHOICES, BUT A RESOLVE TO NEGOTIATE: SITA'S STORY

Mother-in-law says that it would be good if a second boy comes. We thought that since we have one son, if a girl comes this time I will go for an operation, but my mother-in-law says no.

24-year-old Sita is four months pregnant with her third child, and her little girl is just 18 months old. Her first born is a son, aged 4. She belongs to a tribal community from a small village in the Dahod district in Gujarat. She lives in Vadodara with her husband, parents-in-law, brother-in-law and his wife, sister-in-law (husband's younger sister) and two children. Her husband is a driver in Ahmedabad (120 km away), earns about Rs. 17,000 (US $ 206) a month and comes home every fortnight. The other adults in the family usually work as construction workers except for her young sister-in-law, who is studying. This leaves Sita with no help from any of the members of her family for the household responsibilities. Managing mundane household chores and simultaneously looking after her children has not been easy for her. When they are at home, her parents-in-law share some of her workload, feeding and caring for the children, but despite this, her days are quite challenging.

Sita feels controlled by her husband and in-laws. In fact, her husband also does not dare question his parents.

> If we need anything and ask him [father-in-law] for help, he will respond. And we have to obey Papa in every instance. If we have to go anywhere, Papa will accompany us. If we want something, we ask him, and he will bring it for us.

Sita has studied up to Class XII, and feels more fortunate than her parents as her father could only study till Class X and her mother never got an opportunity to go to school. But education has not offered Sita any opportunities or freedom. She is confined within the four walls of her home, doing the same household chores everyday. The only opportunity to go out would be for her to run errands, but her in-laws manage all the outside work. Sita would like to take up a job as a salesperson at the nearby mall but her wishes have been squashed by her father-in-law.

> I was saying that I would go [for a job] at the Mall, but 'his' father [her husband's father] said 'no, who will pick up and drop children from the school? If you would go, who will take care of the children?'

Sita's education has not facilitated her access to reproductive health information. She was unaware of menstruation and what to expect during her periods: her first experience of menstruation left her in fear and confusion. She was in Class XI when she spotted blood on her clothes; petrified at the sight of blood, she asked her mother about it, who dismissed her fears, saying that this happens to ALL women. But more traumatizing than the sight of blood and the realization that this would be a regular phenomenon, was the experience of being treated as an untouchable by her family during her periods. She was barred from touching certain foods, and from cooking and going out.

Post-menarche, life suddenly became very restricted for Sita. It was the end of her innocent childhood, and her mother soon started teaching her how to cook and do other household chores. She realized that she was being moulded to become an ideal daughter-in-law.

> Mother started to teach me household chores, saying that I am 'big' now. She started to teach me how to cook food. She advised me not to smile or laugh too much and not to go out and play.

In school as well, girls were not allowed to go for football practice during periods. They used code language to tell the teacher that they had periods. Then they (the teachers) made us sit aside. We were allowed to go to school but not to play or do any practice.

Young Sita had entered school with the dream of graduating and getting a good job. Soon after she passed the Class XII exams, her dream was shattered when her father met with an accident and her family suddenly faced economic distress. As the eldest child, Sita felt compelled to help and discontinued her education to save costs.

. . . only my father was earning. So as it is, our condition was not good, and then he had a fall and fractured his hand. His operations cost a lot, so I abandoned my education.

Soon after she discontinued her education, her parents got her married. '. . . my parents' wish was that I get married, so I got married'. The girls from her community have no choice in selecting a life partner. Alliances are usually suggested by a relative, after which the boy and his family visit the girl's house to 'see' her. Once the boy approves, her parents and the boy decide on the marriage. The girl's role is merely to serve the boy and the guests tea when they come to see her. The girl's family demands a bride price, sometimes up to Rs. 2 lakh (US $ 2,432). Girls who exercise their choice in marriage are ostracized from the community. Sita remembers how her cousin who married a boy she chose is not accepted in the family even to this day. Lacking the courage to go against her family's wishes, Sita trusted her parents and accepted their decision. Her husband had studied up to Class X.

Sita recalled the events leading up to her marriage. Although her husband lived in the same village, she had never even talked to him until they were married. In fact, concerned about her family's reputation, even after her marriage was decided, she avoided talking to or meeting him until they were married.

Her marriage took place within a month of the visit by her would-be husband and his family. Her parents received Rs. 75,000 (US $ 912) from her husband as the bride price.

Things moved so rapidly that she had no time to think about her future. She received another shock when, within a month of their marriage, her husband announced that they were shifting to Vadodara to stay with his family, who then had lived in another *basti* in Vadodara.

As the eldest daughter-in-law, Sita was encumbered with all the household chores and responsibilities. She found little time for leisure or social interactions.

> It is different. In my mother's home, if I felt like not working after doing some work, I would go out for a walk, sit at my paternal uncle's house, and watch TV for some time . . . but here I have to finish all the work. Here I have to cook for all these people.

With marriage came a host of other restrictions. From wearing a *salwar kameez* in her maternal home, she had to now wear a sari and cover her face with her *pallu* (*laaj*) in the presence of the family elders. Managing the household chores clad in a saree was a tough task. She also felt hesitant initially to ask for things as they were all new to her, but as time passed, she gradually became accustomed to their way of life.

Like menarche, Sita was completely ignorant about sexual relationships when she got married. To date, her husband demands sex when he comes home fortnightly to visit her; she herself has never initiated or expressed her desire for sex. She says her husband does not force her if she is too tired or not feeling well.

Sita missed her periods after four months of marriage. Her mother-in-law took her to a private hospital where her pregnancy was confirmed. Sita was not happy with the news of her pregnancy so soon after her marriage and told her husband about this. Initially, he, too, agreed it would be good not to have a child at this early stage of their marriage. But when his parents admonished him, he refused Sita an abortion and insisted she continue the pregnancy as it was their first child. 'He also wanted the child to be aborted, but mother and father both scolded . . . so. . . .' She had her first childbirth in a private hospital. All the expenses were borne by her husband, including the celebrations, and feasting after the first son's birth. Her parents brought gifts—silver jewellery, clothes, and toys—for the baby as per the custom. Since her pregnancy registration, ante-natal check-ups and deliveries took place in private health facilities, and because the family has an Above Poverty Line (APL) ration card that does not entitle them to government benefits, Sita did not receive any government maternity benefits.[7]

Sita lacked information about conception and contraception as well. She believed that having intercourse during her periods leads to pregnancy. After her son's birth, the nurse from her area gave her a packet of contraceptive pills, but she did not tell her how to use them and for how long, although Sita took one tablet daily. The supply of the tablets ended after two months as the nurse ran out of stock, and Sita did not ask for more. Although she did not use contraceptives, she became pregnant only after two years. Her second baby, a daughter, was also born in the same private hospital, and once again, her husband paid all the expenses. Although Sita wanted to go for sterilization after her second baby, her mother-in-law opposed the idea, insisting that two sons are better than one, especially because the family had farms in their village, and agriculture needs extra hands.

> Son is valued more in our community. Our respect increases with the birth of a son. If the firstborn is a daughter, she gets married and goes away. A son works in the fields. Who will work in the field? When they grow up, the work of farming/agriculture is passed on to them.

Her mother-in-law also added, '. . . girls do not get any share in their father's property; so, it is always better to have another boy in the family'. Her husband was influenced by his mother's reasoning and asked Sita not to go for an operation just then, and she complied, even though she was not happy with the decision: 'I did not say anything when my husband told me to continue with the pregnancy'. Within a year after the birth of her daughter Sita is now pregnant with a third child—against her wishes.

Though Sita still dreams of working in the mall someday, at present she is completely dependent on her husband and his family financially. Her bank account, which was opened to receive her educational scholarships, is no longer functional, and in any case she says she has no use for it as she cannot receive any government benefits. She does not expect to receive a part of her father's property because girls in the community to which she belongs are not given a share.

Despite her experiences of being denied her wishes, Sita is determined to undergo a tubectomy after her third delivery, irrespective of the sex of her third child. She knows that this decision would lead to her facing opposition from her mother-in-law, who wants Sita to have another baby boy. But Sita is determined to stand her ground this time and will negotiate to have her wish fulfilled.

BE THE CHANGE YOU WANT TO SEE: SONAL'S STORY

> We will have a registered court marriage, then I will go and stay with his family. The parents of the bride get a bride price from the bridegroom's family in our community. But I will try my best to convince my parents to not demand any bride price from him or his parents.

Sonal, a 21-year-old young woman, lives in a *basti* in urban Vadodara and works in the branded clothes department at Reliance Mall in the city centre. She adds:

> We need to do things differently, and not support any wrong customs. There is a need for change and that should begin with ourselves.

Sonal has been in a romantic relationship for the last three years. Her boyfriend Rakesh lives with his parents in Vadodara, in a house they own. He is educated, works in a company in Vasna on the outskirts of the city, and earns about Rs. 17,000-18,000 (US $ 207-219) a month. Sonal is acquainted with his family and has visited their house. While they accept their alliance, she fears opposition from her own family and has not yet confided in them.

Sonal's family is against love marriages and she is aware she would have to sever all relations with them when she marries Rakesh. Sonal's mother likes Rakesh but will not support their marriage because he is not from the same community: he is a Darbar, while Sonal is an Adivasi. Sonal saw what happened when her cousin eloped with a boy from within their community: the boy's family had to face their panchayat.[8] The panchayat demanded Rs. 7 lakh (US $ 8,535) from the boy's family as the bride price. The boy was just 21 years old and, distressed by the demands, committed suicide. The younger sister of the cousin who eloped was then forced to marry a boy chosen by her family.

But Sonal is determined to continue with her relationship and will not break it for anything. She is certain she will not go along with her family's plans and marry a boy selected by them and live in a village. The men in her family are very dominating, so she has not revealed her relationship with Rakesh to them. Further, her father has asthma; after treatment for his critical condition in the government tertiary hospital, he is home, but bedridden and on oxygen support with her mother as his caregiver. The family has bought an oxygen cylinder and have it filled when needed.

Sonal is from Dahod, a tribal district in Gujarat. While her mother is her father's first wife, her father married her mother's sister when his first wife could not conceive for quite some time. From the two mothers, Sonal has five siblings, two brothers and three sisters. Her father usually stays with her stepmother and one of Sonal's sisters in Dahod, where they are engaged in farming. Sonal visits them occasionally, but she lives with her mother, two brothers, and two sisters in Vadodara. Her mother and one of her sisters are construction workers.

Sonal studied in a government school till Class X, after which she went for her higher secondary education to a private school but did not pass her Class XII exams. She worked as a salesperson in the D Mart mall for a while before the COVID pandemic, she was on good terms with all her colleagues, and her supervisor was fairly supportive, helping her when she was in need. She was an important earning member of her family then. However, while others in the family supported her, her two brothers did not, and she has bitter memories of that time: 'They are not my brothers but my enemies and want to restrict my freedom'. She used to work late shifts till 10 p.m., and her brothers would follow her to check where she went, but did not drop or pick her up in their auto rickshaw even after late shifts. They tried to force her to leave her job, restricting her mobile phone use and wearing sleeveless dresses, and once created a big scene when they caught her using someone else's mobile. Because she was earning, she had the confidence to stick to her decisions to continue working and open a separate bank account. Her father supported her in these:

> My brother used to accompany me whenever I withdrew money from the bank. But I would not give him the money. I would give it to my parents.

Despite these challenges, Sonal continued working at D Mart, but lost her job during the COVID pandemic. She took on a job as a machine operator in a company that made vehicle radiators on the outskirts of the city. She was promised a salary of Rs. 12,000 per month. However, on the job she met with an accident—her eye was injured. After extensive treatment over three months from three different doctors, her vision was restored, but she could not continue her work after the accident as the heat worsened her discomfort. The manager promised her compensation when she submitted her medical bills, but she did not receive anything. She also did not receive her salary of 51 days.

Working at the Reliance Mall has opened up an entire new world for Sonal. She gets a fixed salary of Rs. 9,500 (US $ 115) and earns incentives of around Rs. 2,000 (US $ 25) if she meets her targets. Her work hours are from 11 a.m. to 8 p.m. and she sometimes has to work different shifts. She is happy at her new workplace, as it is within walking distance of her home, and she has been reunited with many of her friends, some who worked in D Mart, and a few of whom are her school friends.

> I don't know how these six months went by. I enjoy my work here. It's fun.

She grins as she describes how she negotiated with her family on the clothes she could wear. Her uniform at the Reliance Mall comprises branded trousers, a T-shirt, and shoes. When her family learned that she had to wear this uniform, they suggested she go to the mall wearing her regular clothes (*salwar kameez*) and then change into the uniform there. But Sonal said that would be time-consuming, and if she did not reach on time she would be marked late, which would affect her salary. She now goes to work wearing her uniform. About the earlier restrictions on the use of a mobile phone, she laughs:

> I give a considerable amount from my salary to the family. So why should they restrict my use of phone now. I have a smart phone of my own and I use it.

She gives the family her fixed salary (Rs. 9,500; US $ 115) and uses the incentives for herself. The store deposits her salary and incentives in the bank; she has a separate account into which she transfers her incentive earnings.

> I have no unnecessary expenses, and I buy small pieces of silver or gold jewellery. I get satisfaction from these kinds of purchases. As such I do not have any other expenses as I walk to my workplace, have to wear uniform while at work. . . . My family has no reason to object to my separate bank account.

Sonal has told her boyfriend that she will continue working after marriage, as she sees the importance of a job. 'Employment gives one increased knowledge, skill, and earnings'. She wants to buy a bigger house and contribute to the family's income. She seems firm in her decision.

About physical relations with her boyfriend, she told him they would have physical relations only after their marriage. She knows all about planned pregnancies. During her schooling, she was engaged with SAHAJ as a Peer Leader[9] in her *basti*. She learned about sexual and reproductive health rights after engaging with SAHAJ:

> An unmarried couple can have sexual relationship if they are willing to use condom. . . . Sexual relation is not only to have a baby, but for pleasure too. But we need to use condoms.

Sonal's story is one of agency, an agency that results from economic empowerment and the confidence that comes from earning and managing one's finances. The financial autonomy has also boosted the sexual agency she gained from her association with SAHAJ and gives her the confidence to choose her life partner and negotiate critical life decisions including her sexual choices with him.

A VICTIM OF PATRIARCHY: SHEELA'S STORY

24-year-old Sheela's life has been one of contradictions and compromises.

She comes from an Adivasi (indigenous) community from Devgadh Bariya. Her parents, according to her, were traditional, yet she was encouraged to represent her school in sports, ride a bicycle to school, enrol in a higher secondary school and stay in the hostel, and wear jeans and t-shirts. But they strongly disapproved of her interacting with boys, and were not supportive of her when a boy from her school stalked and harassed her on her way to school. They threatened her with dire consequences if she dared to fall in love with a boy of her choice; and she was also discouraged from pursuing a course in nursing after she passed her Class XII examinations.

Sheela was married off to a man chosen by her parents. She wanted to marry a salaried man, but since it was difficult to find one in her community, she agreed to the match even though he worked on construction sites.

She describes her marital family as being well off: they own two three-storied houses, a Scorpio (four-wheeler), and a Bullet (two-wheeler). She had hoped her husband and marital family would support her for further education, and although her parents-in-law gave her permission, her husband prohibited her from doing so. He has studied till Class XII and does not want her to study further:

> My in-laws were supportive of my education after XII but my husband did not agree to it. He has not studied after Class XII hence he did not allow me. He said, 'if I am not studying further, why does she need to?'

Sheela is unhappy and frustrated at this but finds she cannot do anything about it. Determined to put her education to some use, she completed a tailoring course and bought a sewing machine, but she has been confined to sewing or mending clothes for her family.

Other things also changed for Sheela after marriage. She now had to wear a saree and cover her face (*laaj*) in front of the family elders.

> Yes I want to wear (*salwar-kameez*), but I have to wear *laaj*. If I don't have to wear *laaj*, I can wear a *salwar kameez*. . . . He (my husband) asks me to wear *salwar kameez* but mother and father (in-laws) are not letting me wear. When they are not here, I wear *salwar kameez*.

Sheela has to do all the household chores and is berated if her work does not satisfy her husband or the in-laws:

> After marriage all the work was different; at (my) father's place who worked so much? Here I have to do all the work.

Sheela had little information on what to expect after marriage in terms of sexual relations. She had found out about menstruation from her friends at the hostel. She had heard about intercourse from her married friends but her knowledge was superficial. She finds 'getting together' with her husband a little scary but is grateful that her husband respects her wishes for intercourse and 'does not force if she is unwell or tired'.

She admits she had no information about sexual relations, conception, or contraception before she experienced these herself, the lack of which adversely affected her health. She missed her periods two months after she got married. Her mother-in-law took her to a private doctor and her pregnancy was confirmed. Sheela remembers feeling sad at this news—she thought it was too soon after the marriage and wanted to terminate the pregnancy. But her husband refused to allow her to have an abortion, so she continued with her pregnancy:

> After four months of my marriage, I was very upset and feeling sad when I was informed about my pregnancy through the doctor. I wanted to terminate my pregnancy but my husband did not allow it, saying that this was the first baby.

Her pregnancy was not easy, as she experienced severe nausea and vomiting. Her family registered her with a private doctor, but she took medicines from both the private doctor and those given by the *anganwadi* worker. During her antenatal check-ups, the doctor told her that she had sickle cell disease, but she had no information about the disease and what it means for her health. Her husband was advised to undergo a test, and tested negative.

Her first child—a son—was born at the private hospital. Her husband spent Rs. 35,000 (US $ 424) on her delivery. After her delivery she had a copper T inserted, but had it removed after five months, as she was led to believe by her family and friends that it was responsible for her weakness. Within two months of its removal, she missed her periods. Assuming that she was pregnant, Sheela took abortion pills her husband had purchased from a chemist. Six months later, she missed her periods yet again, and the pregnancy-test kit her husband had bought from a pharmacy confirmed her pregnancy. Sheela took abortion pills once again. On both occasions she did not consult a doctor or undergo gynaecological examination.

> I missed my periods within six months of termination of my earlier pregnancy. When I told my husband, he bought a pregnancy detection

strip from the medical store and my pregnancy was confirmed. Then my husband bought abortion pills from the chemist paying Rs. 700, without any doctor's prescription. I took that pills as instructed by the chemist. On the next day, I got my periods with bearable abdominal pain.

Sheela delivered her second child five years after her first child was born. This pregnancy too was difficult, as in addition to severe vomiting, she had severe anaemia. She was given nine iron sucrose injections at the time of her delivery. Yet, Sheela says that her delivery was normal and she did not have any complications after delivery. She was discharged from the hospital the day after the delivery. The doctor gave her no information about postnatal check-ups or contraception. She has not been using any contraceptives, though her menses resumed regularly four months after the delivery.

Sheela is now pregnant for the third time and has been keeping unwell. Fortunately, her mother-in-law takes good care of her, cooking nutritious food and looking after her oldest child.

CONCLUSIONS FROM THE WOMEN'S STORIES

Sita, Sonal, and Sheela are representatives of hundreds of young women of their generation. Their stories reflect the realities experienced by several women from marginalized Adivasi communities, who migrate into cities either after marriage or with families seeking better work opportunities. At several points in their lives, these young women with aspirations for a bright future have been let down by society and systems.

Both Sita and Sheela had to let go of their dreams to pursue higher education, get work and attain financial independence and their own identity to accommodate plans of their families, made without their consent. They were raised in a culture where going against their parents' wishes or selecting their own life partners is unthinkable for young women. Sheela compromised when she married her husband, a construction worker instead of the salaried groom she had always dreamt about.

Marriage was not a happy beginning for them. Sita's husband abruptly moved them from the village to Vadodara city, and Sheela's family did not allow her to pursue a course in nursing. Sita's dream of working in a mall was squashed by her in-laws' expectations that she would be responsible for the household chores and the children. While her husband has no say within the household, he exerts control over Sita in several ways, his demands for sex being one of these.

One also saw the constant tension between life in the tribal areas and the urban environment. Sita's story of completing her high school education in the tribal village, and aspiring to study further, reflects a generation caught between its rural tribal roots and its urban aspirations. She had to suppress her own work aspiration to fulfil the pressures from her mother-in-law to bear sons, because the 'soil has to be tilled and fields have to be sown'. Although the women were from a tribal background, the patriarchal control they experienced is very similar to that experienced by women from other castes.

Both Sita and Sheela feel trapped: Sita because of her controlling marital family and their various restrictions, and Sheela because she was constrained from pursuing further education and engaging in meaningful employment. Another area of control by their marital families is over their reproductive decisions, specifically regarding children and contraception. While both women conceived shortly after their marriages and wanted to terminate their pregnancies, Sita's in-laws did not allow her to do so, and Sheela's husband too prevented her from this.

As Adivasi girls who grew up in villages, Sita and Sheela were able to access higher education because of the special education schemes for tribal areas (such as hostels and scholarships for Adivasi girls). However, exposure to formal education did not help them gain information about their SRH, even though they studied till Class XII. Both found out about menstruation after they had their first periods, had no idea what to expect regarding sexual intercourse, knew little about conception, pregnancy and delivery, and had misconceptions about contraception.

Both women became pregnant with their third child as a result of their lack of awareness about contraception and their lack of autonomy to make personal decisions. The preference for sons is strong in Sita's family and her mother-in-law wanted her to bear two sons before she underwent a tubectomy, so she was forced to carry through her third pregnancy against her wishes. The private doctor whom Sheela's family paid handsomely for her deliveries failed to provide her with crucial information on contraception, which led to unnecessary suffering from unsupervised medical abortions, and a third unwanted pregnancy, even though she suffers from sickle cell disease. The doctor also failed to explain to her the significance of testing positive for sickle cell anaemia. The local nurse/ASHA visited regularly but failed to support her in having a healthier sexual reproductive life.

Sonal stands apart from the other two women on some accounts, despite coming from a similar cultural background. Despite coming from a traditional patriarchal family and experiencing inherent violence she exercised autonomy. She negotiated with her family to continue working in a job that requires her to dress non-conservatively, selected her life partner from another community, and is willing to risk disownment by her family and community for her decision to spend her life with him. She is aware of conception and contraception, and has the agency to negotiate her decisions about engaging in sexual relations with her boyfriend. She attributes her awareness of sexual and reproductive health to her association with SAHAJ during her adolescence.

These stories highlight the failure of the formal education system to sensitize adolescent girls and young women about the sexual and reproductive system. They also point towards limited coverage of school-going adolescents by the various programmes implemented through the *anganwadi*s, exposure to which might have offered the young women an opportunity to gain information about sexual and reproductive health.

The public health system too seems inadequate in responding to their information needs. Sita and Sheela became pregnant within a few months of marriage—before probably being contacted by outreach health workers from the department. Sita was a victim of poor communication on contraception, and a disruption in the supply of contraceptive pills. Despite the state having a programme to detect and provide support for sickle cell anaemia, Sheela was diagnosed with the disease only during her ante-natal check-up and still lacks information on its implications for her health.

In conclusion, Sonal's insight reminds one that the journey to end 'wrong practices', which infringes on the rights of girls and young women, begins with a commitment to change within all. To truly empower them, one must identify harmful practices, challenge patriarchal norms like the bride price in tribal communities, and chart a new path towards gender equality, paving the way for a healthier tomorrow. By creating an inclusive and supportive environment for young people to realize their sexual and reproductive health rights, one can provide them with the means to soar, just like Sonal, enabling them to unleash their potential, assert their rights, and lead lives characterized by autonomy and agency. This transformative journey represents a collective step towards a more equitable and just world for all.

NOTES

1. In 2011, the sex ratio of Gujarat was around 919 compared to the national average of 943; the sex ratios for the SC and ST populations was reported as 931 and 981, respectively (Census 2011).
2. The National Family Health Survey (NFHS) is a large-scale, multi-round survey conducted in a representative sample of households throughout India. To access the latest NFHS-5 data on Gujarat: http://rchiips.org/NFHS/NFHS-5_FCTS/FactSheet_GJ.pdf

3. SABLA is a government-initiated programme aimed at the rural and tribal populations, to provide services for out-of-school adolescent girls related to nutrition, health, and vocation through the ICDS.
4. RKSK is a comprehensive programme aimed at all adolescents. It includes non-communicable diseases, mental health, nutrition, substance abuse, and accidents and injuries. It aims to provide community-based services to adolescents aged 10 to 19.
5. Our field engagement over the last two decades provides several insights into how these programmes are implemented. The next few paragraphs are drawn from the observations of SAHAJ from the field.
6. This is a community-level intervention aimed at adolescents girls aged 10 to 19 years living in the rural areas. It is an add-on to the Mamta Divas which provides fixed day services to pregnant and lactating mothers and children under-five. Mamta Divas, a government of Gujarat initiative, is an important outreach service for adolescents.
7. As per the Pradhan Mantri Matru Vandana Yojana (2017), Rs. 5,000 (US $ 72) is transferred in three instalments to a pregnant women's bank account for the first live birth in the family. The first instalment of Rs 1,000 is paid at the time of registering the pregnancy within 150 days of her last menstrual period, Rs. 2,000 is transferred after six months of her pregnancy, and the third instalment of Rs. 2,000 after registration of the child's birth and completion of the first cycle of her/his immunisation. Additionally, under the Janani Suraksha Yojana (2005), an additional Rs. 600 is paid to a pregnant woman aged 19 and above, from a Below the Poverty Line family or SC/ST family, if she has an institutional delivery in a public health-care facility.
8. These are members of the 'Panchayat' of their community. The Panchayat members are custodians of the community norms and make decisions that are their community members adhere to.
9. SAHAJ conducts programmes for young people in the *basti*s, where local youth are selected as peer leaders, trained and entrusted with training other young people in the community on their rights and entitlements, including sexual and reproductive rights.

REFERENCES

Chakravarthy, V., S. Rajagopal & B. Joshi (2019). 'Does Menstrual Hygiene Management in Urban Slums need a Different Lens? Challenges Faced by Women and Girls in Jaipur and Delhi'. *Indian Journal of Gender Studies*. 26(1-2): 138-59. doi:10.1177/0971521518811174

Ganeshan, Sudhakar. (2020). 'Comparative Analysis of Social Indicators Gujarat vs Uttar Pradesh vs. Tamilnadu vs. Kerala'. *Medium*, 28 August.

George, A.S., A. Amin, C.M. Lopes de Abreu & T.K.S. Ravindran (2020). 'Structural Determinants of Gender Inequality: Why They Matter for Adolescent Girls' Sexual and Reproductive Health'. *British Medical Journal*; 368 -16985 doi: 10.1136/bmj.I6985

Government of India. (2014). *National Youth Policy*. Delhi, Ministry of Youth Affairs and Sports, Government of India.

Government of India. (2023). Census of India. Vadodara City Population 2023 | Literacy and Hindu Muslim Population. Available at: census2011.co.in.

Kotecha, P.V., S.V. Patel, V.S. Mazumdar, R.K. Baxi, S. Misra, M. Diwanji, H. Bakshi, E. Modi, S. Shah & K. Shringarpure (2012). 'Reproductive Health Awareness among Urban School-going Adolescents in Vadodara City'. *Indian Journal of Psychiatry*. *54*(4): 344-8. doi: 10.4103/0019-5545.104821: 10.4103/0019-5545.104821

Mukherjee, Debarati, Shreya Behal & Oommen C. Kurian (2020). 'Investing in Adolescent Health: Harnessing India's Demographic Dividend'. *ORF Special Report No. 115*, July. Observer Research Foundation.

Ninsiima, A.B., K. Michielsen, E. Kemigisha, V.N. Nyakato, E. Leye & G. Coene (2020). 'Poverty, Gender and Reproductive Justice: A Qualitative Study among Adolescent Girls in Western Uganda'. *Culture, Health and Sexuality*. April. 22 (sup1): 65-79. doi: 10.1080/13691058.2019.1660406. Epub Feb 11. PMID: 32045321.

Parmar, H. & U.S. Singh (2021). 'Impact of Health Education on Knowledge Regarding Reproductive and Sexual Health among Adolescent Girls of Anand, Gujarat'. *National Journal of Community Medicine*, *12*(7): 189-93.

Ravindran, T.K.S. & T. Seshadri (2018). 'A Health Equity Research Agenda for India: Results of a Consultative Exercise'. *Health*

Research Policy and Systems'. 16: 94. https://doi.org/10.1186/s12961-018-0367-0

Shah S.P., R. Nair, P.P. Shah, D.K. Modi S.A. Desai & L. Desai (2013). 'Improving Quality of Life with New Menstrual Hygiene Practices among Adolescent Tribal Girls in Rural Gujarat, India'. *Reproductive Health Matters, 21*(41): 205-13. doi: 10.1016/ S0968-8080(13)41691-9

UNDP & NITI Aayog, (2021). *SDG India Index and Dashboard 2020-21: Partnerships in the Decade of Action.* UNDP and NITI Aayog.

Vayeda, M., V. Ghanghar, S. Desai, P. Shah, D. Modi, K. Dave, S. Dave & S. Shah (2021). 'Improving Menstrual Hygiene Management among Adolescent Girls in Tribal Areas of Gujarat: An Evaluation of an Implementation Model Integrating the Government Service Delivery System'. *Sexual and Reproductive Health Matters. 29*(2): 1-16.

Visaria, L. & R.N. Mishra (2017). 'Health Training Programme for Adolescent Girls: Some Lessons from India's NGO Initiative'. *Journal of Health Management, 19*(1): 97-108.

CHAPTER 4

Rural Dalit[1] Women: Experiences from Tamil Nadu

T.K. SUNDARI RAVINDRAN and
P. BALASUBRAMANIAN

THE STATUS OF DALIT WOMEN: MULTIPLE DISCRIMINATIONS

Dalit women in India are at the risk of triple discrimination, ranked bottommost in the traditional caste hierarchy, they face caste discrimination; as women, they face gender discrimination; and being poor, they face class discrimination (International Dalit Solidarity Network and Human Rights Watch 2013).

The Indian Constitution commits itself to the equality of its citizens and to affirmative action to narrow the inequalities between socially marginalized castes and tribes and the rest of the population. However, discrimination and the denial of fundamental rights to Dalit women have been reportedly increasing over the years (Irudayam et al. 2006). The discrimination and violence they encounter at a young age have an overarching effect on their health and well-being. An analysis of secondary data for India found that the average age of mortality for Dalit women was 14.6 years lower than for higher-caste women (UN Women 2018).

Studies in India have shown that women's autonomy, decision making, socio-economic status, poverty, and the extent of gender discrimination they face, strongly correlate with their health, especially their reproductive health outcomes (Yadav et al. 2019). Due to their poor socio-economic conditions,

Dalit women often tend to postpone health seeking and take steps to visit a health facility only in extreme situations. Data from the NFHS-5 (2019-21) found that 61.5 per cent of Scheduled Caste (SC) women faced one or more problems accessing health care compared to 55 per cent of women from socially privileged castes, a statistically significant difference.

Most studies merely present the disparities in sexual and reproductive health (SRH), but qualitative investigations into why and how these inequalities emerge and how and to what extent they affect the lives of marginalized women, are few. Against this backdrop, this chapter presents Dalit women's lived experiences of sexual and reproductive health and rights (SRHR). The stories have been drawn from in-depth interviews with Dalit women as part of a qualitative study by the Rural Women's Social Education Centre (RUWSEC), Chengalpattu, Tamil Nadu, in collaboration with CommonHealth (Coalition for Reproductive Health and Safe Abortion).

SCHEDULED CASTES IN TAMIL NADU AND KANCHEEPURAM

Tamil Nadu is an educationally advanced and industrially developed state. In 2020, its literacy rate was 80.3 per cent (86.8 per cent for males and 73.9 per cent for females). The proportion of population living below the national poverty line was 11.3, far lower than the national average of 21.9 (NITI Aayog 2020), and the average life expectancy at birth was higher for females (72.7 years) than for males (68.6 years) (NITI Aayog 2018). Women's mean age at marriage in the state was 23 years (NITI Aayog 2020). It has good public health facilities, and almost all the deliveries take place in health facilities. Unlike most other states, including Kerala, a little more than two-thirds of the hospital deliveries in Tamil Nadu took place in public institutions (NFHS-5).

Scheduled Castes constitute about a fifth of the population of Tamil Nadu. Dalit movements in the state have a long history and many stalwarts there had started agitations against social oppression even before Independence, initiating different sporadic movements. The 1990s saw the emergence of various Dalit rights groups and of two political parties representing the interests of Dalits—Puthiya Thamizhagam (new Tamil Nadu) and the Dalit Panthers of India (DPI).

Kancheepuram district, in the north-east part of the state has a history of grassroots mobilization by Dalits since the late 1970s. A few Dalit human rights and women's rights organizations emerged in the late 1970s and 1980s which continue to educate Dalit men and women on their fundamental human rights. As a result, Dalit women in the district are more aware of their rights.

SEXUAL AND REPRODUCTIVE RIGHTS AMONG DALIT WOMEN IN TAMIL NADU AND KANCHEEPURAM

As a result of their poor socio-economic status and caste and gender discrimination, SC women in Tamil Nadu experience poor general and sexual and reproductive health outcomes. However, their access to and utilization of menstrual hygiene and maternal health services compares favourably with women of other castes.

SC women and children were nutritionally more deprived than the rest of the population. The NFHS-5 survey for Tamil Nadu shows that the proportion of SC women with low Body Mass Index (BMI) was higher, at 14.3 per cent, than the state's average of 12.6 per cent. Several other micro-level studies also reported that Dalit women in the state suffer from nutritional deficiency diseases (Jaiswala & Valarmathi 2015; Bharathiraja & Hemalatha 2017). About 57 per cent of SC children below the age of five were anaemic (NFHS-5), and the prevalence of anaemia was also noticeably higher among SC women (57 per cent) than others (53 per cent).

Awareness about menstruation and reproductive health was poor among SC girls and women. Based on a survey of 634 SC college girls in four districts of Tamil Nadu, Ravishankar (2017) observed that about 44 per cent had attained menarche without having any idea about it. The same study observed that over two-fifths of the SC students never discussed SRH issues with anyone.

Tamil Nadu's maternal mortality ratio was 54 per one lakh live births in 2018-20, far lower than the national average of 97 (Sample Registration System 2022); one does not have separate figures for SC women. Studies examining the obstetric morbidities of SC women in the state are limited: one study found that more than half (58.2 per cent) of them experienced health problems during their pregnancies (Puthuchira & Athimulam 2014) and that half the Dalit women had faced complications during delivery.

The total fertility rate, which refers to the average number of children that may be expected to be born to a woman in her reproductive period, was 1.78 among SCs (NFHS-5), which is very close to the state's average. However, the infant mortality rate was noticeably higher among them (25.3 per 1,000 live births) than among the other castes (18.6 per 1,000 live births). The SCs also had a higher under-five mortality rate (29 per 1,000 live births) than the average in the state (22.3 per 1,000 live births) (NFHS-5). Thus, SC women in the state faced a higher loss of infants and children.

Despite relatively higher levels of female literacy and economic growth than most other Indian states, the prevalence of spousal violence against women in Tamil Nadu has remained high. The prevalence of physical, sexual or emotional spousal violence for all women was 44.1 per cent in 2005-6, 44.6 per cent in 2015-16, and 36 per cent in 2019-21; in contrast, Dalit women experienced higher levels of lifetime spousal violence, at 52.9 per cent, 54 per cent, and 48 per cent, during 2005-6, 2015-16, and 2019-21, respectively (NFHS-3, NFHS-4, and NFHS-5).

Thanks to Tamil Nadu's good network of functioning government health facilities, SC women and girls report a high utilization of maternal health care and menstrual hygiene products. Nine out of ten pregnant SC women in the state received four or more ANC visits (NFHS-5). Public facilities are the primary source of maternal health care for poor and marginalized caste women. *Anganwadi* centres provide specific support to Dalit women related to maternal health education, health check-ups, and food supplements during pregnancy and breastfeeding. More than 70 per cent of SC women in the state (against 60 per cent among women from the other castes) received special benefits (NFHS-4, 2015-16). An overwhelming majority (83.6 per cent) of SC women delivered their babies in public sector hospitals, far higher than the state average (66.9 per cent) (NFHS-5). A cross-sectional study in Tamil Nadu reported that the probability of a Dalit woman's delivery in a government facility was 2.5 times higher than of non-Dalit women (Balasubramanian 2010). The use of modern contraceptive methods, at 67.1 per cent, was slightly higher among Dalit women than the state average (65.5 per cent). The Government of Tamil Nadu is committed to promoting menstrual hygiene among school-going adolescent girls through the distribution of menstrual hygiene products through government schools. In 2019-21, 98 per cent of all young SC women aged 15-24 years reported using a hygienic method of menstrual protection (NFHS-5).

The women whose stories are narrated in this chapter live in the villages of Kancheepuram (now Chengalpattu) district, where RUWSEC, a grassroots organization working with and for Dalit women, has been working since 1981. The goal of the organization is to promote women's well-being through their empowerment. Its work includes education and information dissemination on sexual and reproductive health rights among Dalits, with a focus on women, adolescents, and young people; service delivery through a clinic; evidence-generation on sexual and reproductive health to foreground the voices of the Dalit community and advocacy for better access to comprehensive sexuality education and sexual and reproductive health services.

The SRH situation of the Dalit women with whom RUWSEC works is very similar to that portrayed above, in terms of their poor nutritional status, general and reproductive health outcomes, and the high prevalence of spousal violence. Access to maternal health services is good, with timely antenatal care and institutional deliveries being almost universal. However, service access varies for other reproductive health problems.

Against this backdrop, the following three stories depict different facets of the sexual and reproductive lives of rural Dalit women in Chengalpattu district, Tamil Nadu. These are stories of women who have experienced extreme challenges to their health and well-being and their sexual and reproductive rights. Gender, class, and caste-based vulnerabilities pose higher risks of health problems playing a significant role in shaping their experiences, with an inequality-blind health system contributing to negative health experiences and outcomes.

'I AM BROKEN. I HAVE NO ONE TO OFFER ME SOLACE': REKHA'S STORY

I have financial difficulties, mental worries, no peace of mind; I don't think I will ever find peace of mind as long as I am alive.

These words capture the current reality of Rekha's life. She is a 29-year-old Dalit woman with two daughters, married to Ranjit, who works as a cook. They live in a thatched hut in a village well-connected by roads and public transportation.

She had not imagined her life would turn out the way it had. She grew up in a loving household with four siblings. Her father was determined that she should be educated, and when she failed in Class X, he arranged tuition classes for her for a year. She passed the exam and joined the higher secondary school, but failed in one subject in Class XII; her father paid the fee for a re-exam, and she completed her Class XII.

Rekha was a bubbly adolescent. She was considered 'bold' because she was comfortable chatting with others, even boys and men. Her parents allowed her to wear jeans and a T-shirt that her uncle from Chennai had gifted her. After completing Class XII, she looked for a job in a 'company', eventually working as a tailor in a large lingerie-producing factory employing around 2,000 workers. Those were happy days.

> I made this one mistake . . . I had a love marriage and am still paying the price for it.

Rekha's husband-to-be, Ranjit, worked as a cook in a hotel near her company. He was from her village and they met on her way to and from work. She developed a 'love relationship' with him. Once when they met at midnight after her shift work, he persuaded her to have sex.

> I did not know . . . that this (pregnancy) would happen. I had no idea about it, and that is God's truth. I thought pregnancy would only happen if we had sex regularly.

A few days after their second or third sexual encounter, Rekha started vomiting and feeling unwell. Her periods were usually irregular, so she did not connect her poor health to pregnancy. However, Ranjit bought her a home pregnancy test kit, and she discovered she was pregnant.

Rekha and Ranjit were scared to share the news of her pregnancy with their families, but eventually both confided in their mothers. Rekha's mother and mother-in-law-to-be took her to the government hospital to terminate the pregnancy. But her condition was too advanced, and a private 'lady doctor' demanded Rs. 18,000 to perform an abortion. Ranjit decided against it and the couple decided to get married. It was a rushed marriage in the local temple; Ranjit's mother and his siblings made the arrangements and met the expenses. No one from Rekha's family attended except her father. Her first baby was over a year old when her parents relented and invited her home for the first time after her marriage.

Ranjit has now become an alcoholic and an abusive husband. During the early years of their marriage, he would support her in sharing in household chores. He would help in washing and drying clothes and bought her a new gold *thali* (*mangal-sutra*) chain. Rekha recalls that when he returned from work late at night, they would talk and laugh about the day's events, and he would console her when his mother scolded her.

Rekha's mother-in-law was unhappy with Rekha because she did not help with the household chores after returning from work and didn't wake up early in the morning after her night shift. Rekha had very little rest; she returned home after midnight when it was the night shift; for the morning shift she had to leave home at 6 a.m. She was not allowed to rest even during her pregnancy.

> I joined work on the 13th day after marriage and worked up to the 9th month of pregnancy. No one asked me, 'Why are you still going to work? Your health is poor. Your feet and face are swollen; how will you pedal the power machine? How will you do the long travel?'

But she had caring friends at her workplace. There, she could eat regularly from the low-cost canteen and received good nursing care from the company clinic. She went back to work after her first baby girl was born. Her mother-in-law was unwilling to take care of the baby and Rekha would bring her baby to the company's crèche.

> From five months, I took the baby with me, come sun or rain. One night, it was raining heavily, and I had just finished my night shift. I had to hold the umbrella, the baby and the bag with the baby's things. The ground was slippery, and I almost fell into a large hole.

Despite all the difficulties she experienced going to work, life was far better when she was employed and had an income. Having to discontinue work because of a severe bike accident was a significant setback in her life. After a couple of years, during which she had a second baby, the company allowed Rekha to re-join work on the condition that she did not get pregnant for at least a year. However, she became pregnant within the year after unsuccessful efforts to have a tubectomy and had to resign.

It affected my financial situation, my development and my self-respect. After that (stopping work), I lost everything. I live like a slave.

Rekha has three children. Her first and second are daughters, aged 9 and 6 years, the third is a son, who would have been 3, but he died in a freak accident at home when he was six months old.

She sought ante-natal care from the local Primary Health Centre (PHC) and ultrasound scans from a local private clinic for all her deliveries, which took place in the medical college hospital. The first was a normal delivery but the second and the third were C-sections. Rekha's second pregnancy occurred within three months of her accident, in which she sustained a head injury and was hospitalized for over two months. She went to the PHC for her delivery, and the entire experience was traumatic:

The nurses asked me to take a deep breath and push the baby out. They also pressed my stomach. I had unbearable pain and shouted, 'Let me go; if you press any further, I will die'. My parents took me to the medical college hospital. There they removed all my clothes and made me stand nude. Then they gave a coat and did the c-section delivery. The baby was injured, with a cut across the face.

After her third delivery Rekha consented to a tubectomy along with the C-section. The baby was a much-awaited boy, and Rekha felt like she had received an unexpected gift, but the infant died when he was only six months old.

She had never wanted to have a third child. After her second delivery, she persuaded her husband to let her have a tubectomy even though both their children were daughters. The hospital asked her to return after her first menstrual period; when she went several months after her first periods, she says:

First, my husband had to sign for the operation. He did not want to, he wanted a boy, and I made him agree. Then we had to give another letter saying our decision was voluntary, although both our children are daughters. Then I had to go and have the blood tests. After that, they said that the doctor who gives sedation (anaesthetist) had not come and that we should come after my next periods. I never got my next periods, I was pregnant.

Her infant son's death was a freak accident. She was cooking with hot boiling oil in the *kadhai* (wok). It was the day of the temple festival, and she came out of her house to see the temple car pass by, and forgot about the boiling oil, which caught fire. In a panic, she grabbed the vessel from the stove and flung it aside to try and put out the fire. Unexpectedly, it fell close to where her baby son lay. He suffered severe burns on his chest and hands, and though they took him to the hospital immediately, he did not survive.

I am not able to bear my sorrow. My memories are torturing me.

Rekha's life turned topsy-turvy after her baby's death. Ranjit had started drinking frequently with his friends after their second daughter was born, and he is now an alcoholic. He is also physically violent, and Rekha has had to seek hospital treatment for her injuries more than once. He has no interest in anything, whether buying things for their home or reroofing the thatched hut, and often says very hurtful things to Rekha:

You killed my son; why should we renovate it (the hut)? Let's live with what we have and die when death comes.

Rekha went home to her parents after one such violent incident, held her father's feet and asked him to forgive and support her. He simply responded with, 'You selected your life partner. What can I do now?'

Amidst the bleakness of her life, Rekha also remembers some moments of unexpected 'enjoyment'. The previous year RUWSEC had held a Woman's Day meeting on 8 March, to which one of their workers had invited Rekha. She participated in various quiz programmes and cultural shows and won many prizes. That day, she could show her talent, her intelligence, it almost felt as if she was back to her early 'company' days, dancing at their events, being the star of the evening.

'I SURVIVED CANCER—AMONG OTHER MISHAPS': MEENAKSHI'S STORY

Meenakshi has been cancer-free for the past 13 years. She is now 54 years old, but she had developed uterine cancer in her late 30s, underwent a hysterectomy and chemotherapy, and won the battle for survival.

Cancer is not the only battle Meenakshi has fought. She lives alone in her marital village and supports herself by selling milk from her three cows. Her one-storey house was built with her earnings and contributions from her brothers. She also leases her two-and-a-half acres of land and earns a small income. Meenakshi was childless after four miscarriages and failed attempts at fertility treatment. Her husband Manohar married again 15 years ago and lives with his second wife and their three children in the company quarters of Manohar's factory. Although still married, Meenakshi does not wear her *thali* because it no longer holds any meaning for her.

Born into a landed and well-off Dalit family and the youngest of eight children, Meenakshi's childhood was happy:

> I used to run around, play hide-and-seek and jump from rooftops. I would hire a bicycle and go round and round the hillock in my village. When someone from the village complained to my brother, he said, 'let her cycle; what's wrong with that?'

Her marriage did not turn out as she had imagined. Her sister and brother-in-law knew the groom's family and even though Meenakshi's brothers were wary of the alliance because Manohar's family was not well-off, the marriage got fixed. Meenakshi did not have the opportunity to see Manohar till the marriage preparations were well underway, and she was disappointed in his appearance because she found him short and thin. But she went along with it because she trusted her family elders' decision.

Life in Meenakshi's marital village could not have been more different from that in her natal one. Manohar and his widowed mother lived in a small, thatched hut that one had to crouch to enter. Rats had dug up the mud floor in many places, and there were swarms of mosquitoes everywhere. Meenakshi hated being there. Even worse, there was often not enough food for her mother-in-law and herself. There was no money to buy onions and tomatoes for the curry to go with the smelly rice from the ration shop, and they would eat it with crushed green chillies. They sometimes had a better meal when they caught fish from the village pond.

Not one to take any situation lying down, Meenakshi brought two buffaloes from her mother's place and started selling milk at a tea shop nearby. Her work with the local organization gave her a modest but stable monthly income. She bought a small piece of cultivable land by pooling her savings and the cash gifts from her brothers. Over the years, she acquired five acres of land, half of which she registered in Manohar's name.

Manohar was a Class VII drop-out at the time of his marriage to Meenakshi. But over the years, he completed Class X, got a technical diploma and moved on to get a salaried job in a company. He kept all his earnings for his educational and other expenses and contributed nothing towards running the household. Meenakshi did not demand any money either; she could find solutions on her own.

We have never had an affectionate relationship, been close, or laughed together.

Meenakshi and Manohar's sexual life began badly. Not knowing anything about sexual intimacy, Meenakshi kicked Manohar away from her on their 'first night'. She continued this for two or three days and he then forced himself on her. Soon Meenakshi realized that her husband was obsessed with sex. There were days when he would call her four or five times a day. Whether it was by the side of a road, the cropland or canal bund, whenever he felt the urge she had to oblige. It came as an extreme shock to Meenakshi when she learnt of his extra-marital relationships with young, unmarried women. When confronted, Manohar would plead, saying he could not live without her. Life went on and nothing changed.

Meenakshi does not think that Manohar was 'violent' even though forced sex was routine, and there were related moments of extreme cruelty. Twenty-five years later, she still shudders to think of the way he raped her the day that she had undergone a Dilatation and Curettage (D&C) procedure following the miscarriage of her first pregnancy within a few months of her marriage.

> I started bleeding heavily, and it was non-stop. I had no one to consult. I informed my husband, but he treated it like a simple matter. I went to a private nursing home alone: they said I had had a miscarriage and the uterus had to be cleaned. I had no money on hand, but I pawned my jewellery immediately and underwent the D&C. . . . I felt that my body parts were being cut and thrown out; the pain was so severe it was as if I was dying. I shouted and screamed from the pain and was very tired after the procedure. The nurse, a woman from my natal village, telephoned my husband and mother. They all came and although my mother wanted me to go to her place, my husband took me home.
>
> He had sex with me the same night. My thighs were swollen, my insides were raw, and I was in so much pain, but he had to have what he wanted. Something happened to me that night, and I was never the same. I think that all my health problems, my three subsequent miscarriages, were because of what happened that day.

After four miscarriages, Meenakshi was advised to try assisted reproduction, which also did not work. As a childless woman, she faced discrimination and stigma even from close members of her family. People considered her presence during *seemantham*, infant-naming, and birthday ceremonies as inauspicious. Seeing young mothers hide their infants' faces when they passed her deeply hurt Meenakshi.

About ten years after her marriage, Meenakshi was diagnosed with uterine cancer. She had noticed that her stomach was bloated, as if she was pregnant. Thinking this could be the after-effect of her many medical procedures, she delayed seeking health care. When she eventually visited a health facility, she was told she had a large uterine tumour and growth in her intestine. The doctors thought surgery would be risky and advised her to spend what remained of her life at home in peace. Meenakshi was not convinced: she consulted several health facilities, willing to die rather than live a bedridden life. A hospital belonging to a private foundation eventually removed her tumours surgically. Six chemotherapy sessions followed; the traumatizing experience of the first session is still fresh in her mind:

I felt like someone had hit my chest with an iron rod. I could not make out whether my eyes were closed or open. I felt like I had fallen off the bed. Somewhere in the corner of my brain, something kept telling me to remove the wires, and I kept shouting out for my niece (who was in the room) to tell the doctors to remove them. I started to scream, and the doctors monitoring the procedure from an anteroom came in and asked me to relax. I don't remember when I drifted out of consciousness, and I woke up in my hospital bed six hours later.

Meenakshi braved six chemotherapy sessions. The post-session after-effects were unbearable, eating and drinking were painful, and the thought of the next session would make her panic. Around this time, Manohar remarried, and Meenakshi also lost her job as a project manager in a women's-centric NGO. She says that, in hindsight, she realized she was mentally ill for some time after the chemotherapy sessions ended.

I would not sleep at night and keep pacing the room, and I would hear people whispering outside and find no one there. At work, I often thought that people were talking badly about me. There were days when I walked to the beach about 2 km from my house in the middle of the night because I wanted to feel the soothing cool breeze against my skin. A concerned co-worker in my NGO encouraged me to join *yoga* and meditation classes. Gradually I started feeling better.

Her husband's health insurance covered many of Meenakshi's medical expenses in the private hospitals, and her brothers paid for the rest. Meenakshi had saved money and gold ornaments and could pay for many of the related expenses. Through the surgery and chemotherapy she stayed with her natal family who took good care of her. But she was sad not to have a loving husband who would support and reassure her. She returned to her marital household sometime after

Manohar had remarried. She lived with Manohar and his second wife for a while, but decided to move out and live alone in the same village.

Meenakshi's life was not merely one of confronting challenges on the personal front. From very early on, she has been a champion for Dalits, especially Dalit women's rights. When she came to live in her husband's village following her marriage, she began to change the course of its history. She persuaded parents to educate their children instead of sending them to graze the upper-caste landowners' cattle; soon, every child aged five was in school. Women were mobilized to tackle everyday problems, like poor roads and streetlights. A few years after her marriage, Meenakshi became a literacy teacher in a local organization dedicated to rural women's empowerment. She worked there for 15 years, rising to be a project manager who developed and managed independent projects. Her achievements include her interventions in cases of intimate partner violence, including a case of femicide, in which she brought the perpetrator to justice. Unsurprisingly, the villagers elected Meenakshi as their panchayat ward member for two terms. Not one to ever say die, Meenakshi continues to be a social activist and leads a federation of self-help groups in her village.

'IF MY HAND AND LEG WERE GOOD, I WOULD NOT HAVE BECOME PREGNANT LIKE THIS': SARALA'S STORY

25-year-old Sarala is now pregnant for the sixth time. She and her husband Franklin live with two of their three children—two boys, aged 3 and 1—in a government-provided group house. Her 5-year-old daughter lives with Sarala's parents. Sarala's family are Christian Dalits belonging to the Vettiyan sub-caste.

Sarala has a physical disability: she cannot stretch or fold the fingers of one hand; one of her legs is bent, and she walks leaning to her left. Franklin, a visually challenged person, is a lay preacher in the local church. Both have disability certificates that give them a monthly allowance of Rs. 1,000 each, their main source of income.

> If my hand and leg were good, I would not have got pregnant like this. I would have worked in some company and moved around freely; I would have money to buy whatever my children and I needed.

When Sarala was a year old, she had a severe fever which left her left hand and leg paralysed. She has awful memories of her childhood. Whenever her parents had work on the land or had to go out, they would place her into a deep sand pit near their house, in which she had to stand for the whole day. Her parents did this to help her as the doctor had advised that standing in sand would strengthen her bones. Sarala could munch on a bowl of puffed rice bowl placed near her, and would be given lunch by her younger sister. She could not use the bathroom till her parents returned and lifted her out of the sand pit. She remembers being sent to Kindergarten (KG) class in the village school but did not study further.

Sarala remembers her menarche as a happy time. She was in a government hostel for children with physical disabilities then. Her father admitted her to the hostel when she was seven. The hostel warden telephoned her parents to tell them about her coming of age. They brought her home and conducted her puberty rituals. Sarala was given a bath with turmeric water and made to stay in a hut made of coconut leaves. Her maternal uncle took care of all the expenses for the celebrations. Sarala's stepmother taught her how to use old cloth as an absorbent. After a year or two, the village *anganwadi* teacher gave her sanitary pads and taught her how to use them.

Sarala moved out of the hostel when she was 15, when her close friend left; she did not want to stay there without her and asked her father to take her home. After that, Sarala would spend her time grazing the goats and protecting the paddy fields from birds and animals. She would leave home soon after waking up and return only around 6 or 7 p.m., very tired, and often fell asleep even before the evening meal.

I decided on my marriage, not my family members. He came in an auto rickshaw to where I was grazing goats and called me. I went.

Sarala met Franklin while she was out grazing goats. He used to visit his relative's house and would sometimes come to the fields to talk to her. She would help him find his way through the fields because he could not see. He gradually took a liking to her, met her father and asked if he could marry her. Her father and brothers refused his proposal because, given his visual impairment, they believed he would not be able to support her financially or physically.

When members of her family did not agree to their marriage, Franklin arrived one day in an auto (rickshaw) to where Sarala was grazing the goats, and she decided to go with him. Her family's efforts at finding her a suitable marriage alliance were not working out. After a week of hiding in the house of her would-be husband's relative, they got married in a church. Her husband's family attended the wedding.

Sarala's married life began well.

He liked me and took good care of me. If I liked something and told him, he would get it immediately for me. I like flowers a lot, and when I ask, he will get them for me and put them in my hair.

But she had a fraught relationship with her mother-in-law, who often took away things her husband had bought for her. She did not allow her to use the bathroom in the house, making her bathe outside the home like the others. What hurt Sarala deeply was the way her mother-in-law humiliated her.

My mother-in-law makes fun of me—calling me *nondichi* (cripple)—she says mean things about me to her friends and laughs tauntingly.

Her mother-in-law's behaviour deepened Sarala's insecurity and this held her back from attending church and formal occasions. 'Who would help her drape the saree? Who would she turn to if the saree came undraped?'

After a few months of her marriage, her husband also started abusing her, often in response to his mother's complaints.

he will listen to his mother's words, question me in abusive terms, and talk in filthy language. He will beat me when he gets angry.

Despite her disability, Franklin expected her to do all the household work. She had to fetch water from the public tap, and had to ask for help to lift the pot to her hip. He did not seem to realize the pain she had to bear. Sarala would cook the food and complete all the household chores and then had to be at Franklin's beck and call:

Get me the towel, fetch me the soap, get me my clothes, give me food, give me *sambar*.

Any delay in her responding to his demands would make him very angry. This behaviour also extended to their sexual life:

If he calls me, I should go immediately. If not, he will curse, scold me, and ask me, 'with whom did you go and roam around that you cannot come soon'. He will even call me a whore, he will not be patient even for a second.

Franklin began beating her if she said she did not feel well. He would insist on having sex even within two months of childbirth. One pregnancy followed another, whether Sarala wanted it or not.

Violence and abuse also contributed to her poor pregnancy outcomes. Sarala lost her first baby after being beaten by her mother-in-law in an argument. She had a lot of bleeding and went to the government hospital for a check-up. When they told her she had had a miscarriage, she was miserable for several months after losing her first child.

A month after her miscarriage, Sarala conceived again. She went to the village health nurse and, on her advice, to the primary health centre (PHC) for monthly check-ups. She was not given any contraceptive advice during her Antenatal Care (ANC) visits but was advised to 'stay away from her husband' after delivery. Sarala gave birth to a baby girl at home, with a nurse conducting her delivery.

Sarala became pregnant again when her daughter was just over a year old, but her pregnancy resulted in a stillbirth due to her husband's violence: she had not been feeling well and hadn't cooked lunch, for which her husband beat her so severely that she bled profusely and went into labour immediately. Her husband took her to the government hospital immediately, but the baby was stillborn. She recalled that the baby boy looked a lot like her husband—his hair, hands, and legs were like his father's.

Her subsequent two babies were sons, both born in government hospitals. She had to depend on her husband to mobilize the money to take her for monthly ante-natal check-ups and the deliveries, sometimes accompanied by her neighbouring *akka* (sister). When there was no money, she would have to borrow to get to the hospital. At the time of the stillbirth, she was taken on a bike to the PHC, and from there on to the government hospital.

> I was bleeding all the way. When the nurses and doctors (in the hospital) saw me, they rebuked me. 'Why did you not come earlier? Could you not have called an ambulance?'

Being blind, her husband could not negotiate the hospital when she was admitted. He left her there and went home, and she had to manage on her own.

Each time she reported a missed period to the village health nurse, the latter would scold her for getting pregnant so often. After her fifth delivery, when her second son was born, she had a copper-T inserted, but it did not suit her. She had heavy bleeding during her periods, lasting for several days, to the extent that she could barely manage to get through the day. Her husband was often away, and she had no one to support her nor any money in hand. Eventually, she went to the hospital with her neighbour's help and had the copper-T removed. She has been told she is ineligible for female sterilization because of her disability, so the doctors advised her husband to undergo a vasectomy. He keeps saying he would but has not done it so far.

Within a month of removing the copper-T, Sarala's periods stopped and she is now four months pregnant. Franklin would like her to terminate this pregnancy with tablets, but Sarala has refused. She wants to give birth to a healthy baby and give the baby to her brother for adoption.

Sarala has not yet gone for any check-ups; she is waiting for her husband to arrange for the money to take her for a scan and for pregnancy check-ups. She wants this to be her last pregnancy.

> I do not want to go on having children; how will I feed them? I cared for all the children without anyone's help and breastfed the babies with the support of just one hand and one leg.

CONCLUSIONS FROM THESE WOMEN'S STORIES

The stories of Rekha, Meenakshi, and Sarala bring home the entrenched nature of gender inequalities and patriarchal control over women's sexuality and reproduction, and how these interact with caste and economic vulnerabilities to shape Dalit women's sexual and reproductive rights and health.

Decades of affirmative action combined with economic and infrastructural growth in Tamil Nadu have made it possible for young Dalit women like Rekha to complete ten years of schooling. The state's industrial policy promotes export-oriented industries, and Kancheepuram district has many factories in special economic zones which employ women with a high school education (Government of Tamil Nadu 2021). For women like Rekha such jobs, despite their precarious nature (see below), offer the possibility of physical mobility and economic freedom.

However, education and employment have not translated into better access to information about sexuality and reproduction for Dalit women like Rekha and Meenakshi. The opening up of opportunities for interaction with the opposite sex without any information about menarche, sexual relations, conception, and contraception expose unmarried young women to the risk of non-consensual sexual encounters and unplanned pregnancies, resulting in forced 'love' marriages.

The economic and educational advancement in Tamil Nadu has not loosened patriarchal control over women's sexuality and reproduction. Gender norms around sexuality strictly censure women's choice of a sexual partner and pre-marital sexual activity, and ostracise women who digress from these norms. Sarala, who chose her own husband, and Rekha, who went through a pre-marital pregnancy, were both ostracized by the community and their own families, leaving them without the much-needed social support. Meenakshi entered into a marriage arranged by her family, without any prior acquaintance with her husband-to-be. While her marriage proved disastrous, she received support from her natal family through all her problems, the social benefit she derived from accepting an arranged marriage. Sexual double standards permitted the men in these stories to enter into pre-marital as well as extra-marital sexual liaisons without any fear of social reprimand.

Gender inequalities marked the women's relationships with their husbands, whether the women had an 'arranged' or 'love' marriage. Their husbands (and in-laws) exercised control over all aspects of their everyday lives, including their sexual relations, conception, and contraception. Non-consensual sex was the norm. In the case of all three women, husbands took no responsibility for preventing pregnancies, and often actively prevented them from using contraception. One sees from Sarala's story that gender inequalities make the experience of living with a disability quite different for a woman compared to a man. Sarala's husband, although blind and unemployed, makes her serve him but does not help her in any way despite his being physically able and strong. She has been forced to go through six pregnancies, because her husband did not allow her to use contraception. Disability did not dampen male control over his wife's sexuality and reproduction.

All three stories recount shocking incidents of intimate partner violence, physical, sexual, and emotional. The extreme and severe nature of the violence caused pregnancy losses, severe injury, and constant emotional distress.

The role of caste in shaping women's general, sexual, and reproductive health is mediated through the poor economic status of women and their having almost no access to or control over the household economic resources. Centuries of discrimination have resulted in most rural Dalit households being landless, poorly educated, and without social networks that could facilitate upward mobility. Higher education is beyond the means of most Dalit women even if they do very well academically in high school, and their income-earning opportunities remain limited to locally available factory-based employment. As one sees in Rekha's case, this means working for daily wages or piece-rate payments, without any job security. Worse still, employment may be contingent on women compromising on their reproductive rights. Rekha had to promise that she would not get pregnant for a year to be re-employed after a major accident. When she was unable to keep her promise, she lost her job. With limited income-earning opportunities, no assets, and no support from the natal family who are themselves eking out a hand-to-mouth existence, Dalit women find themselves trapped in loveless and violent marriages. Meenakshi's story provides a counterpoint, showing what could be possible if women had access to resources; she was able to walk out of her violent marriage and live independently.

The intimate partner violence experienced by Dalit women in this setting may have its roots in their social and economic marginalization. Studies from South Africa on the impact of poverty and economic inequalities on masculinities hypothesize that the origins of violence against women lie in adversity. It is argued that in the presence of widespread material deprivation amidst displays of affluence in unequal societies, men from poor households construct successful masculinities through their ability to access and control women (Wood & Jewkes 2001).

Sarala entered adulthood with compromised health as a result of her physical disability, poor nutrition, and economic deprivation in childhood. While Rekha and Meenakshi did not suffer in the same way, all three were impacted by the lack of adequate nutrition, a heavy workload, and constant stress in their marital homes, which affected their health and well-being. For Rekha and Sarala, intimate partner sexual and physical violence resulted in unwanted pregnancies, pregnancy losses, and delivery complications. Meenakshi experienced severe sexual violence, and subsequently suffered from uterine cancer. The sexual and reproductive health experiences of these women cannot be seen in isolation from their experiences of everyday violence, mental agony, and material deprivation.

All the women sought health-care amidst these challenging circumstances, but unfortunately, the health system too failed them. Rekha experienced disrespect and abuse during her delivery and the denial of timely contraceptive services in a government health facility. Health-care providers failed to prevent Sarala's multiple unwanted pregnancies, by not offering her alternative methods of contraception or counselling her husband to undergo a vasectomy. Meenakshi was able to access private sector services, including for prolonged uterine cancer treatment, because she was covered by her husband's health insurance plan. Few Dalit women would be able to afford private health care for such major reproductive health conditions. The health system is thus blind to gender, caste, and class-based vulnerabilities and does not cater to the less-privileged, especially women.

The lived experiences of Rekha, Meenakshi, and Sarala point to the need for a holistic approach to improving the sexual and reproductive health of Dalit women, one that examines and addresses the root causes of their health problems.

NOTES

1. One has used the terminology 'Dalit' throughout the chapter to refer to women and households of the Parayar caste and sub-castes, but when official statistics or published studies are cited, the term 'Scheduled Caste' (SC) has been used, in keeping with the terminology used by the source documents.

REFERENCES

Balasubramanian, P. (2010). 'Inequities in Access to and Utilisation of Maternal Health Care Services in Krishnagiri and Dharmapuri districts of Tamil Nadu'. Doctoral dissertation. Department of Population Studies, Annamalai University, Chidambaram, Tamil Nadu, India.

Bharathiraja, D. & D. Hemalatha (2017). 'Economic Analysis of Nutritional and Health Status of Dalit Women Agricultural Labour in Cuddalore District, Tamil Nadu'. *International Journal of Management, IT & Engineering*, 7(8). Available at: https://www.ijmra.us/project%20 doc/2017/IJMIE_AUGUST2017/IJMRA-11928.pdf.

Bloom, S.S., D. Wypij & M. Das Gupta (2001). 'Dimensions of Women's Autonomy and the Influence on Maternal Health Care Utilization in a North Indian City'. *Demography. 38*(1): 67-78.

Census of India. (2011). Tamil Nadu, *District Census Handbook: Kancheepuram*, Series 34 Part XII-B. Village and Town Wise Primary Census Abstract (PCA) Directorate of Census Operations, Chennai, Tamil Nadu, India.

Government of Tamil Nadu. (2021). *Tamil Nadu Industrial Policy 2021*, Department of Industry, Chennai.

Government of Tamil Nadu. (2017). *Tamil Nadu State Human Development Report 2017*. Available from https://spc.tn.gov.in/tnhdr 2017.html

Human Rights Watch. (2013). Take Action to Improve Conditions for Dalit Women: Women and Girls Facing Caste-based Discrimination Need Special Protections. Available from https://www.hrw.org/news/2013/06/07/take-action-improve-conditions-dalit-women.

International Dalit Solidarity Network, (2022). *Dalit Women*. Available at: https://idsn.org/key-issues/dalit-women/.

International Institute for Population Sciences (IIPS) and ICF. (2021). *National Family Health Survey (NFHS-5), India, 2019-21: Tamil Nadu*. Mumbai: IIPS.

International Institute for Population Sciences (IIPS) and ICF. (2016). *National Family Health Survey (NFHS-4), India, 2015-16: Tamil Nadu*. Mumbai: IIPS

International Institute for Population Sciences (IIPS) and ICF. (2007). *National Family Health Survey (NFHS-3), India, 2005-06: Tamil Nadu*. Mumbai: IIPS

Irudayam, A., J.P. Mangubhai & J. Lee (2006). *Dalit Women Speak Out: Violence against Dalit Women in India*. Chennai: National Campaign on Dalit Human Rights, National Federation of Dalit Women, and Institute of Development Education, Action and Studies. Available at: http://idsn.org/uploads/media/Violence_ against_ Dalit_Woment.pdf

Jaiswal, A. & Valarmathi. (2015). 'An Anthropological Study on the Profile of Dalit Women in Puducherry'. *International Journal of Scientific Footprints*, *3*(4): 1-14.

Niti Aayog. (2020). *Annual Report 2020-21*. Available from https:// niti.gov.in/sites/default/files/2021-02/Annual-Report2020-2021-English_0.pdf

Niti Aayog. (2018). *Annual Report 2018-19*. Available from https:// niti.gov.in/sites/default/files/2021-02/Annual-Report2020-2021-English_0.pdf

Puthuchira, R. Ravi & K.R. Athimulam (2014). 'Care-seeking Behaviour and Barriers to Accessing Services for Sexual Health Problems among Women in Rural Areas of Tamil Nadu State in India'. *Journal of Sexually Transmitted Diseases*, *8*. doi:10.1155/2014/292157.

Ravishankar, A.K. (2017). 'Empowering Scheduled Caste College Students to Meet Sexual and Reproductive Health Needs in Tamil Nadu: An Intervention Study'. PhD doctoral dissertation, Department of Sociology and Social Work, Acharya Nagarjuna University, Andhra Pradesh, India.

Sample Registration System (SRS). (2022). *Special Bulletin on Maternal Mortality in India 2018-20*, Office of the Registration System, Vital Statistics. Available from: https://censusindia.gov.in/census. website/data/SRSMMB.

Ravindran, T.K.S., P. Balasubramanian & G.K. Mini (2014). 'Inequities in Health in Tamil Nadu: A Study from Dharmapuri District'. In V.K. Natraj & A. Vaidyanathan (Eds.). *Development Narratives: The Political Economy of Tamil Nadu*. New Delhi: Academic Foundation.

Ravindran, T.K.S., & P. Balasubramanian (2007). 'Induced Abortion: A Study of Rural Tamil Nadu'. In Leela Visaria & Vimala Ramachandran (Eds.). *Abortion in India: Ground realities*, New Delhi: Routledge.

Wood, K., & R. Jewkes (2001). 'Dangerous' Love: Reflections on violence among Xhosa Township Youth'. In R. Morrell (ed.). *Changing Men in Southern Africa*. Pietermaritzburg: University of Natal Press. London: Zed Press. pp. 317-36.

CHAPTER 5

Women in Sex Work: Stories from Pune, Maharashtra

SANA QAIS CONTRACTOR and
TEJASWI SEVAKARI

SEX WORKERS IN INDIA: AN OVERVIEW

Sex workers in India are a marginalized, stigmatized, and discriminated group due to the uncertain legal status of sex work in India, and society's moral disapproval. There were estimated to be around 800,000 women sex workers in 2021 in India [National AIDS Control Organization (NACO) 2022]. Owing to the nature of their work and the specific vulnerabilities they face, they are susceptible to a range of sexual and reproductive health problems, including but not limited to unwanted pregnancies, sexually transmitted infections, and other gynaecological problems. Sex workers are also prone to mental health issues as a result of their risk of contracting infections, the social stigma surrounding sex work, and family and intimate partner violence. Therefore, comprehensive and non-discriminatory health-care services are crucial for their well-being. Criminalizing laws of India and negative social attitudes towards sex workers challenge their fundamental human rights, such as their bodily autonomy and their right to choose their preferred work.

This chapter deals with women engaged in sex work in Pune city, who are associated with the organization Saheli Sangh. It attempts to chart their sexual and reproductive health lives, and highlights concerns beyond those that portray them as a 'high-risk' group, as has usually been the case in public health literature.

SEX WORK AND THE LAW IN INDIA

Sex work is pseudo-legal in India, as laws restrict the autonomy of voluntary sex workers. The crime of trafficking for sex work is essentially punishable by both Section 370 of the Indian Penal Code, 1860, as well as by distinctive laws such as The Immoral Traffic (Suppression) Act (SITA), 1956, later amended to the Immoral Traffic (Prevention) Act (ITPA), 1986. Laws administering the right to voluntary sex work in India are unclear. The ITPA 1986 defines sex workers, using the term 'prostitutes', as persons sexually exploited or abused for commercial purposes or for consideration in money or kind. It makes no distinction between voluntary, willing sex work, and coercion, conflating them so both are equally punishable.

The Trafficking of Persons (Prevention, Protection and Rehabilitation) Bill, 2018 adds to the existing laws against trafficking, and assumes that all sex workers are trafficked. Trafficking in the Bill includes forced labour, begging, trafficking women or children for marriage, and administering chemical substances or hormones for early sexual maturity. In addition to detention, the Bill proposes the rescue and rehabilitation of detained sex workers, with no clarity on the status of voluntary sex workers who do not consent to rehabilitation. It also does not contain separate and distinct provisions for children or consenting adults.

The vague nature of the trafficking laws prevent voluntary sex workers from strong negotiation for justice, often leading to discrimination and detention by police officials.

SEX WORK AND SEXUAL, AND REPRODUCTIVE HEALTH RIGHTS

Sex workers are prone to many health problems, owing to the various vulnerabilities enveloping their lives. The absence of a law that overtly decriminalizes sex work is reflected in the lack of suitable health-care policies that could ensure comprehensive, non-discriminatory access to health services for them. Even when such services are available, the clandestine nature of sex work, the social stigma and insensitivity to privacy, and confidentiality obstruct access to these services.

ACCESS TO CONTRACEPTION AND STI PREVENTION

Occupational risks such as unintended pregnancies, unsafe abortions, and transmission of infections underscore the absolute importance of contraception use in the profession of sex work. Through extensive advocacy after the HIV epidemic, awareness and the practice of condom usage among sex workers has increased manifold. Middle-aged sex workers experience greater challenges in negotiating condom use than younger sex workers who have more autonomy, perhaps due to their higher market demand.

Sex workers are generally aware of other methods of contraception, though mostly restricted to sterilization. Apart from the problems of accessibility to condoms, a greater obstruction to safe sex is the refusal by clients to use condoms. Sex workers sometimes fail to insist on condom usage because of more lucrative payments or from fear of violence that may ensue (Ippoliti et al. 2017).

ACCESS TO SAFE ABORTION

In the Indian context, abortion is overly stigmatized and difficult to access for the general population of women, let alone for sex workers. Owing to their high-risk sexual behaviour, sex workers are highly susceptible to unintended pregnancies. A study among 190 pregnant women in Pune showed that 70 per cent of repeat pregnancies among women with HIV were unplanned and unwanted (Suryavanshi et al. 2008). In India, abortion rates among sex workers are far higher than the national average.

INTIMATE PARTNER VIOLENCE

While there are several studies on the commercial lives of sex workers, their interactions with their intimate non-paying partners have a significant impact on their well-being. A study among 1,750 sex workers in north Karnataka noted that 29 per cent of the respondents experienced violence from their intimate partners in the last six months alone (Blanchard et al. 2018); 51.8 per cent of a sample of 998 sex workers in Karnataka had intimate partners, of whom only 22.6 per cent consistently used condoms. There was an 18 per cent decrease in consistent condom use yearly with the increase in the duration of a relationship.

STIGMA IN HEALTH-CARE SETTINGS

Studies show that the quality of health-care services plummets when a sex worker discloses the nature of her profession to a health-care provider (Benoit et al. 2017). The lack of consent and confidentiality in STI testing, delays in or refusing treatment, derogatory terminology, and ineffective treatments are common manifestations of the stigma sex workers face in health-care settings.

Discriminatory attitudes towards sex workers are compounded if they are HIV positive due to the notion that they are vectors of infection. This is a case of 'intersecting stigma' where sex workers are subject to shame for their choice of profession as well as for being infected with HIV [International Center for Research on Women (ICRW), United Nations Development Programme (UNDP) and Skills Strengthening for Industrial Value Enhancement (STRIVE) 2013]. But apart from HIV and AIDS, sexual and reproductive health issues and non-communicable and chronic diseases like hypertension and diabetes remains neglected among sex workers when it comes to awareness, diagnostics, and treatment; cervical cancer, alcohol and drug use, and mental health problems such as depression or anxiety augment their risks and exposure to infections like HIV.

NGOs AND SUPPORT SYSTEMS FOR SEX WORKERS

In India, work with and for sex workers was initiated in the early 1990s around HIV/AIDS awareness and prevention, which was the primary agenda which led activists to focus on sex workers' lives. This led to exploring effective strategies of community engagement—particularly the 'peer education' model—which prepared the grounds for the collectivization of sex workers in India. In the early 1990s, several groups of sex workers were mobilized around their identity as 'workers'.

The purpose of collectivization was to have community leadership and ownership of the programmes and activities, with sustained engagement to recognize and address the various issues faced by sex workers. These collectives helped their community members address and improve their access to health-care services through collective bargaining. The rights-based approach of the collectives definitely empowered and supported sex workers in addressing and solving many of their social, financial, health, and legal issues to a great extent.

SEX WORKERS IN BUDHWAR PETH, PUNE

The women whose stories are shared in this chapter reside in Pune's Budhwar Peth, which is a commercial area housing India's third largest red-light area. It has been estimated that Budhwar Peth, and part of the neighbouring Shukrawar Peth, house about 500 brothels and 4,500 sex workers, with around 150 transgender sex workers residing in one lane.

Pune's red-light area is located in the heart of the city and it has been there since the Peshwa rule, although the form of sex work was different at that time. During the British rule, sex work began to be commercialized in Pune, as it did across India. Pune's red-light area has undergone many changes in the last 40 to 50 years. Between 1980 and 1995 it was run completely by brothel keepers and sex workers from Karnataka, mainly *devdasis*. But this started changing around 1995-6 when the number of Nepali and Andhra sex workers began to rise; and since 2000 one can see a marked increase in sex workers from West Bengal and Bangladesh.

Today, the red-light area consists of women from the rural parts of Maharashtra, Karnataka, Andhra Pradesh/Telangana, Assam, West Bengal, Nepal, and Bangladesh. Girls and women from poor families, mostly from rural areas, with minimum or almost no education come to work as sex workers. There has been a visible decline in trafficking and an increase in voluntary sex work in Pune's red-light area in recent years. Poor financial conditions and the need to earn money for the survival of their families is the main reason for the entry of women into sex work, both voluntarily and through trafficking.

The stories in this chapter document the sexual and reproductive lives of women in sex work, their sexual and reproductive health concerns and health-seeking across their life cycles, and how they relate to sexual and reproductive health in their work and personal lives. They are informed by Saheli Sangh's own experience of working with sex workers and their recognition of the need to explore their health concerns more deeply. While it is true that exploitation exists in sex work, it is also important to note women's autonomy and resistance in practising the trade.

SEEKING LOVE AND FAMILIAL BONDS AS A SEX WORKER: VIMLA'S STORY

Vimla is a 65-year-old woman, born around 1955. Mother to an adopted daughter and a proud grandmother, she resides in Shukrawar peth, a red-light area in Pune. She stopped working as a sex worker when she was about 40 and started working as a peer educator in Saheli 18 years ago. She continues to work for sex workers in Pune's red-light area through Saheli.

Although tricked into becoming a sex worker, Vimla has faced life's challenges squarely and charted her own course as far as she could. She was born into a poor, Dalit family from Bidar, Karnataka. Her family had 10 acres of land; her parents worked on their farm and Vimla also worked there along with her mother. At times her father also worked as a construction worker. She was the eldest among her siblings. When she was six, her mother died during her sixth pregnancy. Her father remarried, as her siblings were ill and there was no one to look after them. But one by one she lost all her siblings, three brothers and a sister, from diarrhoea and other infectious diseases. After her father's remarriage she had four step-sisters and a brother. Vimla would do all the household work and also take care of her younger siblings. She has never been to school and cannot read or write, but learnt to sign her name when she started working in Saheli 18 years ago.

Soon after menarche at the age of about 13, Vimla's father arranged her marriage. Her husband, eight years older, was from a farmers' family and worked on his family's agricultural land along with his father. She had one sister-in-law and a brother-in-law. In her marital home, Vimla did all the household work including taking care of the cattle. It was a difficult life, as she faced domestic abuse especially from her mother-in-law. Several times, she got only one meal to eat in the day. Around nine months after her marriage there was a severe drought in the village. It became so difficult to work the land that Vimla and her husband decided to move to Mumbai and work as daily wage labourers. They worked in Mumbai for almost one-and-half years. Whenever her husband had money, he would eat food outside and drink alcohol, then come home and beat Vimla. There was no one she could speak to as she could communicate only in Kannada. One day they got separated in a crowd and could not find each other. Vimla met someone who spoke Kannada, who assured her he would take her home, but he took her directly to Pune's red-light area and sold her to a brothel. She was 15.5 years of age when she got into sex work. This was about 50 years ago.

For the first six months in the brothel, she was terrified and hid under the brothel keeper's bed when customers entered the brothel. But the brothel keeper never pressurized her to do sex work. The brothel keeper's husband explained to Vimla the reality of sex work:

> as you are in a brothel in a red-light area nobody will accept you back in your family. So, accepting the reality of being a sex worker will help you to sustain here.

Gradually Vimla accepted her life as a sex worker. Her experience with the first customer was not dramatic. 'I had had sexual activity with my husband, so it wasn't unknown to me'.

In the first few months, she had sexually transmitted infection (STI) a few times (including a white discharge and itching), but was completely cured after treatment from a private health-care provider.

After a few years her father came to know of her whereabouts through a relative and visited her, but when he realized she was a sex worker, he suggested she stay in Pune and not come back to the village. Soon after, her father was diagnosed with cancer. She made all efforts to save him, including selling 22 *tola*s of gold given to her by a Marwari client with whom she had her first romantic relationship. But she lost her father when she was around 19; after that she assumed the responsibility of supporting her mother, sisters, and younger brother financially.

At that time, Vimla said, sex workers were not aware about condoms, which were not available in the red-light area. Only customers who were from the army brought condoms. Many sex workers were afraid of using condoms, believing they were used only by those who had a disease, and would therefore avoid customers from the army. She had never used a condom in her entire life as a practising sex worker. But now, because of her association with Saheli Sangh, she has become aware of the different types of contraception methods.

Recalling other differences between 'the past' and now, Vimla mentioned that previously sex workers would avoid working during their periods, whereas today this is not so.

She herself never entertained a customer during menstruation (nor has she used a sanitary pad in her life). Also, previously, most of the customers were decent and dressed properly in a *dhoti* and *kurta*.

In our days, customers chose a sex worker, paid good money, had sex, and left. They only asked for normal (peno-vaginal) sex. But now customers demand dirty sex (anal and oral sex) as they watch dirty movies.

Vimla shared her experiences of her repeated abortions. By the time she was 25 she had had three abortions, all done with the help of a local private medical practitioner who gave her injections to induce an abortion. She never conceived after the three abortions; the medical practitioner had told her that because of repeated abortions at a young age her uterus had been permanently damaged, so she would be unable to conceive. Whenever a sex worker became pregnant, they would be sent to the same medical practitioner. The brothel keepers insisted that the sex workers in their brothels seek services exclusively from him, and they paid for this. The brothel keepers and sex workers did not seek health services from government hospitals due to the fear of stigma and ridicule. Also, at the time many minors were engaged in sex work in the red-light area, which would criminally implicate the brothel keeper.

Hamare zamane mein sachha pyar hota tha (In our days we had true love).

Vimla talks about the romantic relationships in her life as experiences of true love. When she was around 18, she had her first romantic relationship with one of her regular customers, which continued for a few years. Since he was from a good family, Vimla believed that he ought to get married and settle down. She convinced him to marry a woman from his own community and helped him start his married life. He continued to visit her regularly right until his death three years ago, and even helped her through a financial crisis.

When she was 30 she fell in love with another customer who married her and took her away from the red-light area. Her 'husband' was already legally married, so their marriage did not have any legal status. After her marriage Vimla started working as a maid in the home of a rich family in Pune. After a few years, she and her husband came back to live in her husband's inherited house in Shukrawar Peth, a red light area. Vimla continues to live there even after her husband's death.

Vimla never became pregnant after her third abortion. When she was around 50 she adopted a daughter, although the adoption was not a legal one. She had started taking care of the little girl after her mother, who was a close friend of Vimla's, died from AIDS-related complications. This form of adoption is very common among sex workers. Her daughter is now married and Vimla has a grandchild. She still carries a deep hurt and feels used by her natal family who have not accepted her despite benefitting from her financial help.

Presently Vimla is working with Saheli Sangh as a board member. Given her advanced years, she is not actively working as a peer leader but looks after some of the day-to-day logistics in the office and mentors new community leaders.

'I HAD A TUBECTOMY AT 25: I DIDN'T WANT ANOTHER UNPLANNED PREGNANCY': RESHMA'S STORY

Reshma is 45 years old and from Kathmandu, Nepal. She gave up sex work almost 18 years ago and now works in Saheli Sangh as a peer leader and caretaker in their transit home for the children of sex workers. She has lived in Pune for the past 25 years and currently lives with her partner of 15 years in a rented house outside the red-light area. Her son and daughter are married.

Reshma faced physical and mental violence right from her childhood. Her family was very poor and her parents had to work very hard for their survival. She worked on the farm; hunger was a constant, and she and her friends would often steal fruit and food from neighbouring farms and hide in the jungle to eat, to avoid being punished by members of her family.

Reshma has never been to school. Girls were never sent to school, and were expected to do the household work, since they would eventually marry, leave their homes and not support their parents. Her elder brother, who studied up to Class VII, was the only one in her family who had gone to school.

Reshma was married when she was 8—her father arranged her marriage and she was completely unaware she was married. In her maternal home, she worked very hard: for an 8 year-old it was very difficult to cook food for 15 to 20 people. Reshma spoke about how girls and women in Nepal had to do all the household work as well having to work in the farms.

She had four mothers-in-law: 'More wives meant more labourers in the family!' One day, one of them beat her so badly that she ran away to her natal home. Her father had a huge physical fight with her in-laws, who filed a police complaint against him, and he was sent to jail for six years. Reshma's mother held her responsible for this and as a result ill-treated her. Reshma ran away again to a friend who she used to call 'sister'. The friend assured her she would find her a job in a big city in India. She brought her to Mumbai and sold her to a brothel.

Reshma had not yet reached puberty when she was sold into sex work. She had to do household work for about six to seven months till she reached menarche, and soon afterwards was forced to start sex work. She was completely unaware of what this entailed. Language was also a barrier, since she understood only Nepali, her mother tongue.

After staying in Mumbai for six to seven years, Reshma returned to Nepal, but came back to India soon afterwards as her mother had passed away and her father had remarried. She lived for some time with a man who had promised to help her. This was an abusive relationship which resulted in a pregnancy and the birth of a baby boy. Reshma moved to Surat city for a few months and then to Pune.

After coming to Pune, she handed her child to a caretaker outside the red-light area and continued doing sex work. After two years she got into a relationship with one of her regular customers, who then became her regular partner for eight years. Her second child, a daughter, was born from this relationship. The relationship ended when the man married and left Pune for his native village. Reshma never saw him again and does not know if he is still alive.

When she became pregnant for the first time, she was around 17 or 18 and was not even aware of her pregnancy. She was not much older during her second pregnancy; she said that she treated both pregnancies very casually. When her first child was just a year and a half, Reshma became pregnant for a second time because condom use among clients was almost negligible. She did not want to have another baby as her son was still very young, so a friend, a fellow sex worker, helped her get an abortion. She went to the private clinic of a doctor who was the preferred health-care provider for sex workers at that time. He gave her an intravenous injection and saline, bleeding started, and the abortion occurred. Reshma says she was mentally prepared for the procedure and did not have any complications subsequently. She had two induced abortions, and took oral contraceptive pills for several years after her second child. She underwent a tubectomy at the very young age of 25, because her menstrual cycle was irregular, and she did not want to live in fear of another pregnancy.

Talking about the availability of contraceptives when she first entered sex work, Reshma said that only mala D (oral contraceptive pills) was available then, and that clients did not use condoms. Sex workers would get an abortion from a private clinic for only Rs. 300 to 500.

When Reshma started living with her current regular partner 15 years ago, she thought of having a child with him. She went to the hospital to find out if her tubectomy could be reversed, but changed her mind because of the uncertainty around relationships such as hers.

How long will a man provide support? One must live life on one's own terms.

She has now reached menopause and battles with restlessness and depression, which she associates with menopause.

Reshma was very particular about condom use during sexual intercourse to prevent HIV infection.

I have slept on an empty stomach on many days—but never entertained a customer without a condom.

She had undergone HIV testing several times to confirm she is not HIV-positive. Three years ago, she was diagnosed with diabetes and started taking medicines.

Reshma had wanted to get out of sex work all her life, and she succeeded in getting away without help from any man. She now works with Saheli Sangh as a board member and active peer leader. She is very active in the Sexual and Reproductive Health (SRH) sessions and in providing SRH services to women in sex work.

'I AM MORE IN CONTROL OF MY LIFE NOW THAN BEFORE I ENTERED SEX WORK': PRIYA'S STORY

Thirty-two-year-old Priya has been engaged in sex work for almost 15 years. She lives in a rented house outside the red-light area with her current partner. Renting a house was difficult for a single woman. She takes care of her previous partner's school-going daughters who live in a hostel near Pune.

She comes from a town near Pune city, where she lived with her parents and three siblings. Her father collected scrap and her mother worked in a hotel earning a decent living. She loved going to school and was good in sports and maths. When she was 16, her father died in an accident; her mother was severely traumatized and stopped working. The family's financial situation worsened and Priya had to discontinue her studies. She and her elder brother started working for daily wages in scrap collection.

Priya had a boyfriend when she was in school. She recalls how their romantic relationship evolved: friends since childhood, they began developing special feelings for each other when they grew to be adolescents. They grew physically intimate and enjoyed the intimacy. They met once or twice a week, used to kiss each other, and have sex once or twice a month. 'Those feelings were totally different', she reminiscences. They were planning to get married and start a life together.

If he would have been alive, I would not have taken up sex work.

Sadly, Priya's boyfriend died in an accident. She was devastated at the time, little realizing that things would become a lot worse. Used to having irregular menstruation, Priya did not realize that she was pregnant when she missed her periods. When she realized after four months, she went to a clinic seeking an abortion. The doctor was abusive and did not help her. A friend who came to know that Priya was pregnant suggested that she takes five tablets of Crocin, but that did not result in an abortion. By the time her mother realized that Priya was pregnant, she was over five months pregnant and so an abortion was not possible in any clinic.

Fearing disapproval from the community for her pre-marital pregnancy, Priya and her mother left their town and moved to Mumbai. Priya worked collecting scrap, and also started working in a liquor shop. It was very difficult, as she worked hard day and night. Her only aim was to save money for the birth and her child's upkeep. Unfortunately, she also started using *gutka* due to the influence of her peers at work, and became addicted to it.

Around 12 days after she returned home from the hospital after her delivery, Priya asked for the money she had saved. Her mother's partner, an alcoholic, had squandered it all. Offended by Priya's demands, her mother beat her and threw her out of the house.

It was raining heavily and Priya had no place to go. She reached a railway station, stayed there for the night and next morning boarded a train without knowing where it was headed. The train reached Pandharpur, a famous religious place in Maharashtra. There she stayed outside the temple with her child. A police constable in the area started giving her food and milk for the baby. The local small shop owners started asking if she had come to do *dhandha* (sex work); she did not know what they meant. The police constable gave her Rs. 300 and put her on a train to Pune.

Thereafter, Priya travelled from place to place by train and started begging. Eventually she returned to Pune railway station and started living with some young pickpockets, who looked after her and her six-month-old baby. One day when she was sick and sleeping, her baby was abducted. She lodged a police complaint, but never found her child again.

During this time, Priya had fallen in love with one of the pickpockets. He had a daughter, but he did not work, so he could not support either Priya or his daughter. Survival was difficult. On the suggestion of one of her friends who was a part-time sex worker, Priya rented a room and started sex work. Entertaining customers was initially very painful for her, both physically and emotionally. For the first six months, she hardly had one or two customers a day, but she gradually became used to the work and began having 4-5 customers a day.

Her partner harassed and abused her physically and sexually, and took all the money she earned from sex work. Not able to cope, she left and started staying in the red-light area. Her next partner was a married man, who took good care of her, and they even started living together. Priya continued her work as a sex worker while he worked as an ambulance driver. She listed the man as her husband in all the legal documents. They lived together for six years, until he died of liver failure. Priya still misses him a lot.

Talking about the birth and loss of her child, Priya says,

> After childbirth my entire life was ruined, I started begging and living on the streets for six months. When my child was kidnapped and I never got him back, I started behaving like a vagabond, staying anywhere, eating anywhere, sleeping anywhere.

She never became pregnant again; the doctor had told her she has 'a swelling in her uterus'. She did not want to have another child, so she did not take any treatment for the condition.

Priya feels that she is more in control of her life now than she was before entering sex work. She takes care of her previous partner's daughters and currently has a regular partner. She always negotiates and insists on condom-use with all her customers and ensures that her prior and current partners undergo HIV tests regularly. She has herself tested for HIV regularly and is HIV-negative.

Her brothers are aware of her profession, but she no longer cares about their views and visits them whenever she wants. She has no more regrets:

> I do not bother about anything in life! I can live life on my own terms as a sex worker.

CONCLUSIONS FROM THESE WOMEN'S STORIES

Although the category of women in sex work has been of interest to public health researchers for several decades, their vulnerability has been seen largely as one that predisposes them to particular health problems—such as HIV/AIDS, STIs, unwanted pregnancies, and multiple abortions. However, the case studies presented in this article reveal a much richer tapestry of their sexual and reproductive lives, which underlies both their vulnerability as well as their agency.

COMPOUNDING VULNERABILITIES AND 'CHOICE'

First, the case studies demonstrate the vulnerabilities resulting from the intersecting axes of power—gender, caste, and class, especially—that dictate the women's choices and their ability to overcome their circumstances. Throughout their lives, one sees the impact of gender norms and patriarchal oppression. They face sexual and domestic abuse from childhood in their natal families, early marriages without any decision-making power, and subsequent mistreatment in their marital homes. Their reasons for leaving their homes and taking up sex work are also often related to gender—such as a premarital pregnancy or facing extreme abuse. The vulnerabilities they face upon leaving home are strongly rooted in gender—the constant unwanted attention of predatory men, being cheated easily due to the lack of support, struggles for survival especially when they have young children, being sold into or entering sex work, and eventually, due to the stigma attached, being left with no choice but to remain in sex work.

While this is not explicitly articulated in the case studies, the fact that two of the three women were from the lower castes suggests that caste can make a woman more vulnerable to drift into sex work. Another important aspect was being a migrant: one of the women was from Nepal; she had run away and, with few other options, took up sex work in India.

While two of the women were sold into sex work and therefore had no choice, one 'chose' sex work as a way to survive. The women largely maintain that they chose their customers and decided when they wanted to engage in sex work, but this 'choice' is undeniably a complicated one given that their options were very limited. This was their only source of income: once they entered sex work, structural factors and societal stigma further ensured that their choices remained restricted.

The profession of sex work, although seen as 'work' for the purpose of this study, is further rooted in gender and caste discrimination, and capitalizes on the vulnerabilities of the women and girls engaged in it. The fact that it is criminalized, as it is seen as being 'immoral', enables the exploitation of the women—by customers, by brothel owners, as well as by the police. Women do not have much say in the 'rules' followed by the brothels and red-light areas. They accept these and work towards gaining more autonomy as they become more experienced. While engaged in sex work, even though they have breached the stated limits of 'morality', they continue to perform gendered roles—such as caring for their families and providing for their children, often at the cost of their own well-being. Despite having financial autonomy, familial acceptance is still difficult to attain.

SEXUAL AND REPRODUCTIVE HEALTH PROBLEMS

In terms of control over their reproductive autonomy during sex work, it appears that the women used whatever means were available to ensure contraception—but these were was not always appropriate. Reshma for instance got sterilized at a very young age because her menstrual cycle was irregular and she did not want to become pregnant inadvertently. Even though their work involved a high risk of unwanted pregnancies and sexually transmitted infections, before the onset of the HIV epidemic, women reported almost no consistent use of or access to modern contraceptives. However, when they had unwanted pregnancies, they were usually in a position to get an abortion, although whether this was safe or not is not known.

Despite living in the city of Pune, where public health services are available and physically accessible, the sex workers appear not to use the public health system at all. They prefer private providers—usually a particular provider in the red-light area referred to by the brothel keeper. This is because of familiarity as well as the fear of facing stigma and discrimination at a public health facility. Further, despite being an at-risk group, there seems to be very little outreach to the sex-worker community with SRH services. The HIV epidemic brought some attention to the issue of STIs, and the use of condoms appears to have increased over the years according to the women. But it is also clear that they use condoms largely for STI prevention, and typically, only with non-regular partners. This provides some insight into how the health system views sex workers—typically as carriers of a disease that needs to be curtailed. But it does not tackle the myriad other health issues they face from being engaged in sex work (especially the difficulties of access to contraception abortions, and STI prevention and treatment), or their needs as women—i.e., for maternal health, mental health, etc.

REDEFINING 'FAMILY' THROUGH UNCONVENTIONAL RELATIONSHIPS

There is a certain redefining of traditional relationships evident in all three narratives, both with romantic partners as well as with children. The women's relationships with their children varied depending on their circumstances. In some instances, children were sent away and in others they stayed with their mothers. But in all situations, women took great pains to ensure that their children were provided for, and even if their own families was unaware of or unwilling to acknowledge their work, they took on the financial burden of looking after their children. Having a child also made the women more vulnerable and, in at least one instance, the woman entered sex work to ensure survival for herself and her child, and in another, the woman's child was abducted. Adoption of children is also a common practice among women in sex work, as one saw in the case of Vimla, who at around 50 adopted a girl and raised her as her own. The adoption was not legal—she started taking care of the child after her mother, her close friend, died from an AIDS-related complication.

As in their relationships with children, the women's relationships with their romantic partners were also clearly unconventional, born out of constrained choices in difficult circumstances. Apart from formal marriage, the women were engaged in various long-term stable romantic relationships, sometimes in the nature of a marriage. The nature of these relationships was varied and the women recalled them with both horror as well as fondness. Some relationships were abusive and exploitative; in other instances, they were much more loving and even gave the woman the status of marriage, even though in some cases the men were already married or were encouraged by the sex worker herself to get married to a 'respectable' woman.

Vimla developed two such long-term relationships, one when she was young and the other when she was older. In the first, the man continued to stay in touch with her, visit her, and even help her out financially. Her second relationship was with a man who promised her a 'marriage-like' relationship, took her out of the red-light area and gave her his name. Many of these relationships defy convention and labels, but are nevertheless deeply significant and have played a very important role in the women's lives. They signify a certain resistance to difficult circumstances, where the women have attempted to make the most of situations that they found themselves in.

RESISTANCE AND AGENCY

While gender and other axes of vulnerability place women in a position of dire powerlessness, their stories also present continuous efforts at posing resistance to their circumstances, thereby defying the 'victim' stereotype that is often associated with sex workers. At every stage, they find a way to make space for themselves and survive. Even while they are engaged in sex work, the women have made repeated attempts to leave or find other sources of sustenance. Those who have become reconciled to their work, have resisted being victims and have in fact been active participants in creating a new life for themselves. The financial resources they garnered as they grew more experienced in sex work also gave them greater autonomy in spending their money. While the women have expressed resentment and sadness at finding themselves alone in their old age, they continue to have independence and sources of sustenance. They have drawn solidarity from others, from their children, and also from being part of collectives like Saheli Sangh.

REFERENCES

Benoit, C., M. Jansson, M. Smith & J. Flagg (2017): 'Prostitution Stigma and Its Effect on the Working Conditions, Personal Lives, and Health of Sex Workers'. *The Journal of Sex Research*. doi: 10.1080/00224499.2017.1393652

Blanchard, A.K., S.G. Nair, S.G. Bruce, et al. (2018). 'A Community-based Qualitative Study on the Experience and Understandings of Intimate Partner Violence and HIV Vulnerability from the Perspectives of Female Sex Workers and Male Intimate Partners in North Karnataka state, India'. *BMC Women's Health*, *18*(1), 66. doi:10.1186/s12905-018-0554-8

Gangoli, G. (1999). 'Unmet Needs: Sex Workers and Health Care'. *Indian Journal of Medical Ethics*, 7(3): 92.

International Center for Research on Women (ICRW), United Nations Development Programme (UNDP) & Skills Strengthening for Industrial Value Enhancement (STRIVE) (2013). *A Global HIV Stigma Reduction Framework Adapted and Implemented in Five Settings in India. Summary Report*. International Center for Research on Women (ICRW).

Ippoliti, N.B., G. Nanda & T.D. Mastro (2017). 'Meeting the Reproductive Health Needs of Female Key Populations Affected by HIV in Low- and Middle-income Countries: A Review of the Evidence'. *Studies in Family Planning*, *48*(2): 121-51.

Javalkar, P., S. Isac, R. Prakash, T. Raghavendra, G. Sudhakar, C. Kundannavar, M. Das & P. Bhattacharjee (2015). *Stigma and Discrimination among Female Sex Workers: Learnings from a Pilot Project in North Karnataka, India*. Bangalore: Karnataka Health Promotion Trust (KHPT).

National AIDS Control Organisation (NACO). (2022). *National AIDS and STD Programme Phase V (2021-2026): Anchoring the National Response Towards Ending the AIDS Epidemic*. New Delhi, Ministry of Health and Family Welfare, Government of India. Available at: https://naco.gov.in/sites/default/files/NACP_V_ Strategy_ Booklet.pdf

Pai, A., M. Seshu, M. Gupte & VAMP. (2014). *Status of Sex Workers in India*. Available at: http://tbinternet.ohchr.org/Treaties/CEDAW/Shared%20Documents/Ind/INT_CEDAW_NGO_Ind_17395_E.pdf. Accessed 12 February 2017.

Suryavanshi, N., A. Erande, H. Pisal, A. Shankar, R. Bhosale, R. Bollinger, M. Phadke & J. Sastry (2008). 'Repeated Pregnancy among Women with Known HIV Status in Pune, India'. *AIDS Care*, *20*(9): 1111-18. doi: 10.1080/09540120701842753

Vijayakumar, G., S. Panchanadeswaran & S. Chacko (2019). 'Sex Work, Marginalization, and Activism in India'. *Archives of Sexual Behavior*, (48): 1969-72. Available at: https://doi.org/10.1007/s10508-018-1384-3

Weiner, R., M. Fineberg, B. Dube, et al. (2018). 'Using a Cascade Approach to Assess Condom Uptake in Female Sex Workers in India: A Review of the Avahan Data'. *BMC Public Health*, *18*(1): 897. July 20. doi:10.1186/s12889-018-5842-6

WHO. (2005). *Violence Against Sex Workers and HIV Prevention*: Information sheet. Violence against women and HIV/AIDS: critical intersections. Department of Gender, Women and Health, Global Coalition on Women and AIDS Information Bulletin Series, Number 3.

Harcourt, C. & B. Donovan (2005). 'The Many Faces of Sex Work. Sexually Transmitted Infections', *81*(3): 201-06. doi:10.1136/sti.2004.012468

CHAPTER 6

The Adivasi Community: Silent Struggles—Unveiling the Lives of Sabar Tribal Women in Khordha, Odisha

V.R. ATKURI and BIJAYALAXMI RAUTARAY

THE ADIVASI COMMUNITY IN KHORDHA, ODISHA

The Adivasis (original settlers) or tribal communities are perhaps the most deprived and exploited group in India today. Communities that lived in harmony with nature and in a sustainable manner with the environment in a forest economy have been systematically deprived of their dwellings and their sources of food and livelihood and displaced in large numbers in the name of development. Many have been forced into poverty. Across all the development indicators in the country—income, education, health, mortality, literacy levels, nutrition—the tribals fare the worst (NFHS-5). Since they traditionally live in hilly or mountainous forested areas, access to health and health-care services, as well as access by health-care providers, is difficult.

Tribals form 22.8 per cent of the population of the State of Odisha (Census of India 2011). Their sex ratio in Odisha (1,029) is higher than among the general population in the state (979). And although it is assumed that tribal communities show relatively lower levels of gender discrimination, the *Economic Survey of India 2011-12* indicated that the Gender

Development Index (GDI) in most tribal districts in Odisha is poor.

For example, an alarming 67 per cent of tribals in Odisha are poor. The largest proportion are labourers (45 per cent), while 38 per cent are cultivators, and the rest have other occupations. In the poorest quintile, labourers form the largest group (54 per cent), while in the richest quintile, the largest group (58 per cent) are engaged in other occupations, such as self-employed non-agricultural occupations, or as regular wage earners (Parida undated).

The stories in this chapter focus on the sexual and reproductive life histories of Sabar tribal women living in Khordha district of Odisha. The Sabars have been labelled one of the 'Particularly Vulnerable Tribal Groups' and are scattered across many states. In Odisha only a few Sabar groups in the interior hill areas retain their tribal customs and habits, while the rest have been Sanskritized to varying extents. The Sabars living in Khordha district migrated there many generations ago and do not retain any tribal identity: their language and customs, as well as their religious practices are identical to the rest of the people in Odisha.

The proportion of tribal population in Khordha district is relatively low, and therefore it has not been designated a tribal district, nor does it have any tribal blocks. The Sabars in Khordha, therefore, do not benefit from the special programmes targetting the tribal areas. Additionally, many of them are not recognized as tribals and are denied a 'tribal' certificate. One reason for this is that in some government records, instead of Sabar or Sahar, their names were recorded as *Kabari*, or *Saara*, which are not tribal names. Hence they are deprived of the benefits tribals are entitled to: they have no access to government schemes for tribal children, such as free education in *ashram* schools, or reservation in higher education and jobs. Those who do have the 'tribal' certificates are better off economically.

Though tribal women typically have a relatively better status than their counterparts from other communities, Sabar women in Khordha bear the consequences of Sanskritization: their community in Khordha has unfortunately adopted some of the patriarchal practices from the Hindu communities, and gender inequality is more marked among them than it is in other, less- Sanskritised tribal groups. This means that there are restrictions on women's movement and clothing after menarche; they have no say in who they marry or when; son preference is common; and domestic violence is prevalent.

Thus, the Sabar women of Khordha are more deprived than tribal men—suffering all the deprivations that tribal men do, and further being subject to the gender discrimination emanating from their adoption of the Hindu religion and customs. Their lives are a seemingly unending cycle of poverty and malnutrition, amidst cultural constraints. They live in scattered geographical locations across a mainly hilly terrain. They have low literacy rates and lack information on issues related to their health and physical well-being. They live isolated lives and have limited interaction with women of other communities, with the exception of the female frontline health workers at the village level. Little is known of what their lives are like,. what they go through from childhood to adulthood, and what they feel about their lives.

It is necessary, therefore, that their voices be heard. This document is an attempt to bring their voices and experiences of sexual reproductive health and rights to the attention of the public and policy makers.

The following three stories depict different facets of the sexual and reproductive lives of Sabar women in Khordha in eastern Odisha.

LIVING LIFE ON HER OWN TERMS: OR NOT? MEENA'S STORY

Meena, a Sabar woman in her thirties, lives with her husband and five-year-old daughter in Aranga village in Khordha district. Her husband Mithun works as an agricultural labourer and also does other casual labour, though he does not find work every day. She, too, works as an agricultural labourer. Her in-laws live in a separate house with one of their granddaughters in the same compound as Meena, as do her husband's brother and his family.

As one of four siblings, she and her two sisters were controlled by their brother and beaten for anything he considered as disobedience. This included visiting friends or playing outside the house. It was only after she was old enough to collect firewood or work as a labourer did she get some freedom to be away from home and meet other people. She had no knowledge of her body or of sexuality. When she got her periods, her grandmother taught her how to manage them, but she had to make changes in how she dressed after that. She had no say in who she married; her marriage was arranged with someone she did not care for.

She recalls what she felt on the seventh night of her marriage when her husband first touched her:

> I started crying. When he grabbed me, I remembered my paternal home. I thought, 'my brother will get angry if he gets to know about this. Why is he holding me?' I cried. He left me alone that day.

She did not like her first sexual experience after marriage and refused sex for four years. Her husband did not force her to have sex, but after four years left home and went to work in a brick factory. According to Meena, Mithun would work, drink alcohol, and stay with friends.

However, she worried about what others would say about her not having a child. She was afraid of sex, but was anxious too:

> I thought to myself, 'Although I will be fine (without sex), this man may say something to others'. I had some fear in me. I thought, 'If anyone gets to know about it, they might judge me. They may ask what kind of woman is she.' I got intimate with him due to the fear of what people would say.

She was taunted by her in-laws and neighbours for not having a child, and she also began to long for a child of her own. When her husband returned after two years, they started living together as husband and wife, and she conceived. This was six years after her marriage. She had no knowledge of the signs of a pregnancy, and was anxious when her periods stopped. She had regular ante-natal care and delivered a girl baby normally in the district hospital. But subsequently, she developed severe anaemia and needed a blood transfusion to survive; she also developed asthma.

She now lives in a state of anger and worry. Though her husband would like another child, she does not, as she finds it difficult enough to bring up one child.

> We are unable to raise this one child properly. We are unable to give her nice clothes. What would we get by having another baby? It's all about raising the baby. This girl alone has given us a very hard time. She constantly says, 'I want this, I want that; I won't eat this, I won't eat that'.

She is angry with her husband who is now an alcoholic and does not help her, not even in errands like fetching groceries. She worries about how she will educate their daughter. Though they were given a house under the Indira Awas Yojana, it was severely damaged in a cyclone, for which they got no compensation. As a beneficiary of the Ujjwala Yojana she was given a free cooking gas connection, but cannot afford the refill. Work as a labourer, both for her husband and herself, is sporadic. She feels she has no happiness in her life. Still, she manages to maintain her identity and individuality in a conservative, patriarchal society.

A DIFFICULT LIFE: SUKANTI'S STORY

Sukanti Behera, an agricultural labourer, lives with her husband and three daughters in a village in Khordha district. They live in difficult circumstances: as an agricultural labourer she earns a daily wage of Rs. 200, while her husband earns Rs. 300. With forests diminishing rapidly, there is less and less firewood available for collecting and selling. She feels that they do not have a proper house, unlike her grandfather's large house which had four rooms. That house and land have been sold by her male cousins and she got some share of the proceeds.

There is no National Rural Employment Guarantee Scheme (NREGS) work in her village, but she has an Aadhar card, a ration card, and a voter ID; the family does not have a (state-government issued) health insurance card. The few benefits entitled to her family through government schemes have remained on paper. She has a bank account in her name which she opened for the Ujjwala scheme to receive a gas cylinder. She has never refilled the cylinder, as they could not afford to pay for it and her husband 'sold' the cylinder to another family, who refill it periodically, with the subsidy amount being credited to her account. A toilet pan was placed (under Swachh Bharat Mission), but there is no pipe or pit attached so they cannot use it.

Sukanti's childhood was also impoverished, and she and two sisters were forced to start working from a young age. In her words,

> What would we eat if we did not work? We were from a very poor family, and our parents were old. Even having two meals a day was very difficult. When we were a little older, our parents told us to go and collect firewood. I tell you, even with a small amount of money like 10 annas, I would run to buy rice and salt, otherwise we would have been starving.

Only their youngest sister was sent to school. Sukanti had no say in choosing her life partner. She was married to a cousin-by-marriage, someone she did not want to marry, as he was poor too and lived in a dilapidated house. A dowry of Rs. 5,000 was demanded and given; the money was what her father had kept from Sukanti's earnings. Sukanti is no longer in touch with her family now, which is a matter of sorrow for her.

She was ignorant about sex when she married, and her first sexual experience after marriage took place after being bribed with chocolates. At the time she wanted to run back to her natal home, but she stayed out of fear. She recalls what happened to a woman from her village:

> She was from our village. After marriage, she left her in-laws' house and returned to her natal house. But her brothers were furious, as they felt that by returning she had damaged their reputation. They had her beaten and killed.

She felt that as a woman she had no choice but to stay with her husband and cater to his sexual needs.

Her first three deliveries were at her in-laws' home. All three girls were breech born, delivered at home, but none of them survived. During her pregnancies she had to continue to do all household chores, including carrying water uphill to their home. She conceived within four months of losing the first baby and continued to work throughout. After losing each of her babies she would resume work immediately as she worried about what others would say:

> If I hadn't worked then they would say—just because her child died she is sitting at home and we should work? Why?

Subsequently, on a friend's advice, she went to her parents' home for her subsequent pregnancies. She had three more children—all girls again, who were born normally at home, and are alive and well. In her parents' home she got enough rest, and only did some light chores during her pregnancy.

She feels very sad about her three lost children. She also faces comments from other women in the community:

> My wish was for four children, including one son and daughter. I saw first a daughter, then another. . . . Daughters were born, but none lived, and people began to say things like, 'Her face is inauspicious'. My sister-in-law says, 'Who will see her face?' (She had no child, but said this when I also didn't have any). Even now they call me 'anthukudi' because I don't have a male child.

Her youngest child is now about 12, and studies in Class VII. Sukanti's periods ceased just after the delivery of her last child, but she did not consult a doctor to find out why. She has never practised contraception, nor has she discussed this with her husband, and they stopped having sex after her menopause. According to her, there is no point in sex now as she cannot conceive. She also feels old—her oldest daughter has attained menarche and she imagines it would be odd for her and her husband to still be having sex.

Her main concern is her financial status and the fact that they have no home. Her husband's house where they live, collapsed completely after the tropical cyclone Fani, and they have no money to rebuild. Due to the COVID pandemic and lockdown, work is hard to get. Their one-room house has no door. Several young men wander around their locality, and with alcohol consumption very common, she is concerned for the safety of her daughters in a house that cannot be locked. Her daughters sleep inside and she and her husband sleep outside the house.

Post-script: Since the first contact the authors had with her, Sukanti died following a COVID-19 infection. Her oldest daughter set herself on fire when she was not given the money she demanded for clothes and jewellery. She was admitted to the hospital with 80 per cent burns and had to remain there for three months. She is back home now, but with memory loss and cannot speak properly.

'HE THRASHED ME, WE FOUGHT OFTEN': KINU'S STORY

Kinu Pradhan, a Sabar woman from Khordha district, is unhappy and sad about her life, saying she has had a difficult childhood and married life.

> In my life I have faced difficulties in my paternal home as well as in my in-laws' home. I haven't got happiness anywhere. . . . From my childhood I had to work. I was the one who purchased various things for the house. Then I got married and came here but I could not buy anything here, either. As long as my parents-in-law were alive, I enjoyed my life and felt happy. After they died, the sadness returned to my life. . . . Even after doing so much for the family, my husband does not appreciate me.

Kinu lives with her five children and husband in a half-constructed hut, and works as a construction labourer. Her husband is a seasonal migrant labourer who goes to Chennai for work, for three or four months at a time. He works at different jobs—road construction, in a factory, or wherever he gets a paid job. She is the one who takes on the responsibility of borrowing money for essential things like house repairs.

This has been a recurring theme in her life: Kinu started working early when she realized that her father was the only earning member, as her brothers did not work. Describing her experiences while growing up, she is not sure at what age she attained menarche, only that she thought she was wounded and bleeding till her cousin told her otherwise. She could not understand the changes in her body, like the enlargement of her breasts. When her aunt refused to talk to her about it, she asked her brother and father, for which she was scolded by her aunt: '"No, it's not right to ask anyone about this". After that I did not talk to anyone about it.'

Though she liked a non-tribal boy who returned her feelings, she did not have the courage to elope with him when he asked her. Her marriage was arranged with someone from her own community. When she went to his house after the wedding she found that it lacked facilities she was used to in her natal home, like proper water supply and electricity.

In her marital home she was 'taught how to behave'. How to walk slowly, how to remain covered with a veil in the presence of men other than her husband. She resented the veil as she could not then see properly and would often stumble into things, once venturing into the space of her brother-in-law.

When her husband first touched her after marriage, she was scared and ran away to sleep with her mother-in-law. A few weeks later her husband told her that men marry only to have sex and if she refused him, he would think she was involved with another man. Her first sexual experience was a violent one. Her husband tied her hands behind her with a towel and forced her to have intercourse. She felt terrified and suffocated and shouted for help but no one answered;

she also experienced severe abdominal pain. After a few times, she got used to intercourse and sometimes even enjoyed it.

Her first pregnancy happened soon after her marriage, and she had her babies in quick succession—her first three children are now 15, 13 and 12 years old. After the ASHA explained the rhythm method to her, she and her husband began practising it, though he does so reluctantly. Her fourth and fifth children are now 6 and 3 years old. The Auxiliary Nurse Midwife (ANM) asked her to have a tubectomy, but she refused, thinking that it would make her weak, and since her husband does not work and earn enough, she has to take care of the family.

Of her five children, the first and last were born at home. For her first delivery they did not have the money to go to a hospital; in fact, her father-in-law was in the process of going to mortgage the house for a loan when her baby was born. She had ante-natal care for all five pregnancies. The ASHA accompanied her for her hospital deliveries. After each child-birth, she would rest for 21 days before she resumed domestic chores, and then go back to agricultural labour when her child was a year old.

Her husband beats her when he is drunk, especially for not doing what he says, and for lending money to others.

> When I have some money, I lend it to other women who need it. If I have money and don't give it to another woman in need, where will she roam around (for help)? He would say, 'and what about you? . . . you are also roaming around to borrow money. . . . Are you their servant?' Saying this, he would beat me.
>
> When people ask, I would say 'We were having a Dubulu fight,' and hide my injuries and hurt with my smile.
>
> The shopkeeper uncle would ask, 'Kinu, has Mohan beaten you with the stick today?' I would say, 'He thrashed me, we had Dubulu fight.' Then he would tell everyone.
>
> My husband would thrash me to the point that I would lose consciousness, and then would cry later (as he felt sorry). He would go on beating me in a fit of anger. When I would not come home or prepare food, he would cry and scream and cook food himself, and then call me to have food.

He has not been beating me as much since our eldest daughter attained menarche. The beatings have reduced to some extent. I told my daughter about that Dubulu fight. I said, 'Your father had beaten me like this.' She would say, 'Are you finding it funny, as you are telling everyone that you had a Dubulu fight?'

In my life I have faced difficulties in my paternal home as well as in my in-laws' home. I didn't find happiness anywhere.

CONCLUSIONS FROM THESE WOMEN'S STORIES

Odisha is the state with the third largest tribal population and has the most diverse indigenous communities found in the country. Tribals in coastal districts like Khordha, living in isolated pockets retaining virtually none of their original culture and social habits, are probably more disadvantaged than those in interior, designated scheduled areas which have specific provisions for development. So, in spite of the efforts made by the government for affirmative action for tribal communities, the Sabars in Khordha district continue to remain marginalized. Their Sanskritization and the denial of their tribal identity has worsened the status of their women who are already facing the adverse effects of poverty. While they can access most government schemes provided for people below the poverty line, the last-mile connectivity for the delivery of benefits is missing.

These three stories show how marginalization interacts with gender to mould women's precarious reproductive pathways. They face the adverse outcomes of the lack of education, heavy workload, low wages, and limited means of livelihood, along with patriarchal control of their sexuality and reproduction.

Neither Meena, Sukanti nor Kinu had any knowledge of their bodies or of sexuality while they were adolescents. Menarche and sexual intercourse were milestones they faced without being prepared or being ready for them. In fact, Kinu was actively discouraged from seeking any information about changes in her body. None of them were given a choice about who they married—this was decided for them. They faced patriarchal control—Meena's brother controlled where she could go or who she could play with; Sukanti remained with her husband fearing she would be killed if she returned to her parents' home; Kinu faced a lifetime of violence from her partner—right from the time of her first sexual intercourse, to regular beatings through her life.

Apart from poverty, the women's lives are marked by pressure to conform to societal norms. Access to health care is limited because of poverty—Sukanti had all her babies at home even when she had lost her previous babies. They face various pressures—to have babies, to have sons or be condemned as infertile and a bad omen—as well as intimate partner sexual and physical violence. Amidst all this, they resist, retaliate, negotiate, compromise, and survive.

Poverty is a common theme through these stories: the families barely managing to make ends meet; the need to keep working since work is irregular; the husbands are alcohol-dependent. Though they are eligible to apply for government schemes, poor implementation of these programmes means that they do not actually receive the benefits.

Thus toilets are built, but are incomplete; gas cylinders are provided but the refills are unaffordable; and women have access to the ANMs, ASHAs and AWWs, but they lack basic information on their bodily processes like menstruation, pregnancy, childbirth, and contraception. Government programmes, such as the self-help groups formed through the AWCs, are not there in their section of the village. Most people are unaware of the health insurance scheme run by the state government. As tribals they are kept apart from the general population, but as they are not officially recognized as tribal they are deprived access to government-provided facilities, and their children are deprived access to affordable education and secure jobs. Even this denial seems arbitrary: those who were fortunate enough to have their names spelt correctly get the 'tribal' certificate; others from the same family with a differently spelt name are denied it.

The stories of these women are of multiple deprivations and denial of rights—social, economic, reproductive, and sexual, as well as the right to health care.

REFERENCES

Government of India. Census Commissioner, Ministry of Home Affairs. *Primary Census Abstract, Odisha:* Available at: http://censusindia.gov.in/Tables_Published/H-Series/houselist_ main.html

Government of Odisha. (2012). *Economic Survey, Odisha, 2011-12*, p. 262. Available at https://pc.odisha.gov.in/Download/Economic_Survey_2011_12.pdf

International Institute of Population Services (IIPS). (2021). *National Family Health Survey 5, 2019-21*. National Family Health Survey 5 Odisha. Available at: http://rchiips.org/nfhs/NFHS-5Reports/Odisha.pdf

Parida, S.P. 'Tribal Poverty in Rural Odisha'. *The Tribal Tribune*, 5(3). Available at: https://www.etribaltribune.com/index.php/volume-5/mv5i3/tribal-poverty-in-rural-odisha

CHAPTER 7

Sexual and Reproductive Justice for All: What Would it Take?

RENU KHANNA, T.K. SUNDARI RAVINDRAN and SUBHA SRI B.

This book shares the stories of the sexual and reproductive pathways of women who experience multiple marginalizations, in their own voices. The protagonists are young women (both married and single) from different parts of India—some from the Adivasi [including Particularly Vulnerable Tribal Groups (PVTG)] and Dalit communities, and include sex workers and women who migrate to cities either after marriage or in search of better work opportunities. The layers of vulnerability they face are a result of structural exclusions due to caste, class, gender, ethnicity, age, geographical location, and stigmatized occupations like sex work. In these stories one sees how women's life situations, external contexts, and specific events have differential influences on their sexual and reproductive health across their life stages. While vulnerabilities because of class, caste/ethnicity, age, and occupation compromise their health and well-being, gender power inequalities constitute the fulcrum around which their sexual and reproductive health and rights revolve. An insensitive health system exacerbates their negative health experiences and outcomes. Looking at the world from the perspectives of women on the margins can change one's understanding and practice (Indira 2020) of what it takes to achieve sexual and reproductive justice.

In the following sections, the key emerging themes on the pervasive influence of their marginalized status and gender power inequalities on women's sexual and reproductive health and rights are summarized. In the first section below, the emerging conceptual framework for understanding the factors that shape the sexual and reproductive justice of women living on the margins are presented. It draws on the women's stories to elaborate the various elements of the conceptual framework. The second section reflects on how the women's narratives have enhanced one's understanding of the factors influencing sexual and reproductive justice and the implications for knowledge-building and social action.

THE EMERGING CONCEPTUAL FRAMEWORK: THE FORCES SHAPING WOMEN'S ACCESS TO SEXUAL AND REPRODUCTIVE JUSTICE

Looking at the world from the perspective of women living on the margins has enabled an understanding of the complex interplay and cumulative effect of multiple factors resulting in the denial of sexual and reproductive justice to women. Below, a conceptual framework emerging from the women's stories, is presented.

Denial of Human Rights and Social Justice

The denial of human rights and social justice results in the marginalization and exclusion of specific population groups. For Dalit and Adivasi groups, this is the result of the denial of economic, social, and cultural rights for centuries, resulting in their disproportionate representation among those living in poverty, without access to land or adequate housing, being illiterate or having limited education and having casual or even precarious employment and low wages. In 2021, five out of six persons living in multidimensional poverty in India belonged to the Dalit or Adivasi communities (UNDP & OPHI 2021). Historical marginalization, in turn, increases the probability of migrating in search of livelihood, often resulting in added vulnerabilities. For women, patriarchal social norms and patriarchal control in their households combine with marginalization and social exclusion, with far-reaching consequences on their life opportunities, health, and well-being.

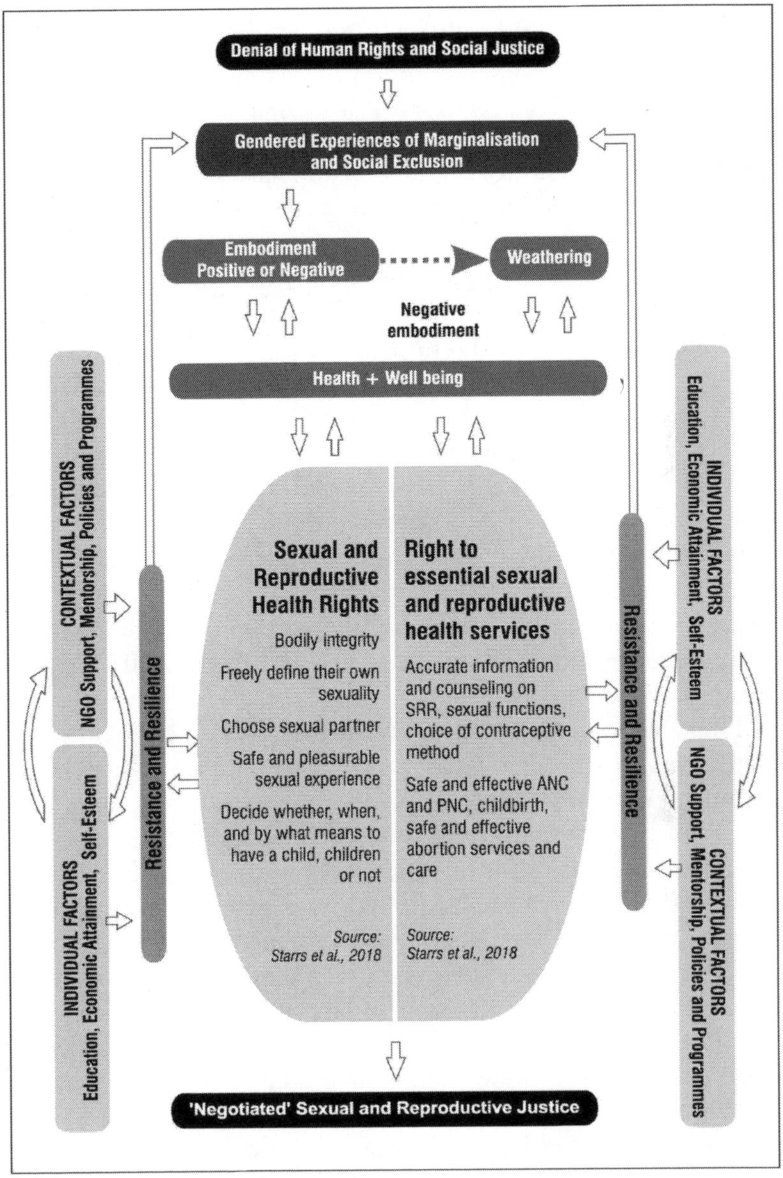

Source: Developed by the Authors, 2024.

Figure 7.1: Factors Influencing Marginalized Women's Access to Sexual and Reproductive Justice

Gendered Experiences of Marginalisation and Social Exclusion

The Role of Gender in Material Deprivation

The women whose stories have been shared in this book are all 'living on the edge'. Precariousness is a recurring theme in the stories: precarity due to inherited abject poverty as a Dalit or Adivasi woman, and also from the impact of natural phenomena like cyclones, man-made conflicts like communal violence, and the COVID-19 pandemic. Material deprivation, poverty affecting their dreams and aspirations, and adverse events that push families over the brink of indebtedness are undercurrents in all the stories.

Food insecurity and hunger in childhood are features of many of these women's lives and continue through adulthood. Gender differentials in the quantity and quality of food allocated to adults and adolescents across all income levels are well established in India and are likely to be particularly stark in low-income households (Arnold 2009; Aurino 2017; Patel et al. 2013).

The women who narrated their stories lived in poor housing conditions—in overcrowded houses in congested urban slums or mud houses with thatched walls in rural settings. Personal safety and security were a source of concern to them and their families, resulting in restricted physical mobility which limited their opportunities for education, employment, and social interaction. The lack of basic amenities at home meant many arduous hours of domestic work for girls and women because of the gender division of labour in their homes.

Limited household resources, distributed in favour of males, often prevent girls and women from pursuing higher education and force their entry into the labour force, including as sex workers. The feminization of poverty is seen in the women's narration of starting to work early in life and bearing the burden of their families and children even after marriage. At the same time, their husbands often drank away all their earnings.

Being Dalit, Adivasi, or a migrant means not only having limited economic resources but also limited social capital, and thus exclusion from access to many opportunities. All the three women in sex work had been denied schooling, and two of them belonged to socially excluded castes, thus highlighting the role of caste in women's marginalization.

Poverty also shapes how disability is experienced. Sarala, who had a physical disability, suffered from neglect as a child because her wage-labouring parents had to leave her unattended when they went to work. She discontinued her schooling after a few years and was engaged in grazing cattle as a young girl. Her lack of education proved to be a significant disadvantage in later life when she found herself trapped in an abusive marriage.

As seen in the case of Dalit women who experienced severe forms of intimate partner violence, poverty and social marginalization can play a significant role in the spawning of violent masculinities. Although there are no Indian studies examining this relationship, studies from Sub-Saharan Africa have demonstrated, through men's narratives, that unemployment, everyday misfortunes, and socio-economic marginality drive poor urban men to establish their self-esteem and male worth through intimate partner violence against women (Izugbara 2011; Jewekes et al. 2015).

Patriarchal Control Over the Lives of Marginalized Women

Being a woman triples the burden of marginalization and exacerbates their exclusion resulting from constraints imposed by unequal gender power relations in society.

The exercise of power within gender relations is manifested in restricting women's autonomy along various dimensions, such as education and employment opportunities, freedom of movement, dress, and enjoyment of sexual and reproductive rights (described in a subsequent section). It is wielded by fathers, fathers-in-law, brothers, mothers, mothers-in-law, and husbands. While the nature of control experienced by the women in these stories is similar to that of Indian women in general, their marginalized social location has a major impact on the consequences of such control on their lives. Control over women's freedom is especially evident in the case of young unmarried women. Although Sonal (Vadodara) worked in a mall, her brothers, whom she thought of as 'enemies', dictated a dress code for her, prevented her from using her mobile, monitored her movements by following her, and tried to force her to leave her job. Mothers are also expected to keep their unmarried daughters 'under control' and ensure they do not bring dishonour to the family through behaviour that does not conform to socially accepted gender norms. The exercise of power by mothers-in-law is mentioned in many of the women's stories. They expected their daughters-in-law to take complete responsibility for domestic chores, which, given the poor housing conditions under which they lived, involved many hours of arduous labour.

Unequal power relations between the women and their husbands have many facets. In its most benign form, male power was expressed as deciding what one's wife could or should do. All the wives, including Sarala who lived with a physical disability, were at the beck and call of their husbands. The men controlled household spending and determined how much their wives could have. Many husbands also supported their parents' control of their wives, while others tacitly supported their mother's inconsiderate demands and even outright violence on their wives.

While such controlling behaviours are themselves manifestations of economic and emotional violence, physical and sexual violence by intimate partners is a recurring theme in almost all the women's stories (such as Sarala's experience of violence by her husband). This is a clear example of how intersectionality plays out, with male privilege overriding the disadvantages of disability and caste position.

Sexual violence also manifests as non-consensual sex, including in the case of the women who experienced pre-marital pregnancies. Some of the stories around sexual violence are horrific and heartrending, such as Meenakshi's narration of being raped by her husband on the day she underwent a D&C procedure after her miscarriage.

Embodiment and Weathering

The consequences of women's gendered experience of marginalization combined with the patriarchal control of their lives are seen in the 'embodiment' by women and the weathering of their bodies.

According to Krieger (2005a), who conceptualized 'embodiment', 'Bodies tell stories about—and cannot be studied divorced from—the conditions of our existence'. Simply put, embodiment is about how the social and physical environments within which we live become embedded within our biology. Societal arrangements of power, privilege and opportunity—and conversely, of disadvantage, marginalization, and exclusion—are reflected in our bodily experiences of health, and well-being or of ill health and trauma. Inequalities in health are 'embodied expressions of social inequality' (Krieger 2005b). In the stories presented in previous sections, one sees how the historical and cumulative stress of being a PVTG, Dalit, poor migrant, or sex worker living in a particular context is carried in the women's bodies and results in poor reproductive, mental, and general health.

Related to embodiment is the concept of 'weathering'. The weathering hypothesis (Geronimus 1992) states that populations who face racial discrimination in terms of social, political and economic marginalization experience an early breakdown of physiologic systems, which leads to premature ageing. Weathering can thus be understood as the embodied consequence of the inequalities of power, privilege and opportunity, leading to disparities in health outcomes.

Embodiment and weathering are important determinants of poor sexual and reproductive health, and the violation of sexual and reproductive rights; they also mediate timely access to quality sexual and reproductive health services. In turn, poor sexual and reproductive health and poor access to services—manifested as repeated pregnancies, unsafe abortion, maternal morbidity, pregnancy and child loss, infections, and everyday violence—are embodied in and further accentuate the process of weathering.

Sexual and Reproductive Health Rights

Most of the women made their sexual and reproductive debut in a state of compromised health. A childhood spent in poverty and hunger, with poor housing inducing insecurity, financial difficulties, lack of autonomy, and discord in the natal or marital households, underlies their lack of physical and mental well-being. The women's stories are replete with accounts of anxiety, anger, sadness, frustration, and disappointment. Many of them experienced a feeling of 'aloneness' when shouldering familial responsibilities amidst their precarious livelihoods. One of the women experienced a pregnancy a few months after sustaining a head injury from a road traffic accident. Women's multiple marginalization and poor health status circumscribe and permeate their experiences of sexual and reproductive health and rights.

Sexuality and Sexual Rights

The lack of knowledge and information about sexuality stands out in the women's stories. This reflects societal taboos and silence especially around female sexuality. Women's marginalization also limited their access to other sources of information, such as the print and visual media and the internet. Lack of information on sexuality often translated into a violation of their other sexual rights as well, including non-consensual sex and their inability to experience sexual pleasure. This lack of access had life-altering consequences for some of the young women, such as their entry into sex work, ostracization by their parents and a hurried marriage.

Marriage is not a choice but an imperative for all the women. Sexual activity and sexual relationships outside of marriage are prohibited, and women's sexuality has to be controlled until marriage allows socially sanctioned sexuality for reproduction. Most of the women avoided premarital sexual relationships because of societal sanctions. Those who transgressed these norms paid a heavy price.

Most were denied the choice of their husbands (and hence, sexual partners). Arranged marriages were the norm, with the women abiding by the choices made by their elders. Whether arranged by their elders or chosen by themselves, marriage was not a happy experience for most of them. Those who went against social norms and chose their husbands, experienced the denial of parental support through their difficult lives, a high price to pay while living in poverty. On the other hand, 'obedient' daughters and sisters could count on support from their parents and siblings.

It seems possible that gender norms around sexuality may be stringently followed in marginalized communities. For people living on the margins, social approval may ensure social support, often their only resource in times of adversity.

Reproductive Health and Rights

Pregnancy was not a rosy experience for the women, who were poorly nourished, shouldered a heavy workload, steeped in anxieties and, at times, in poor physical health. Those who worked outside their homes had to continue working in both places till late in their pregnancies. For women in sex work, like Reshma, pregnancy was often an occupational hazard.

Poor pregnancy outcomes—miscarriages, stillbirths, infant deaths—are rarely prioritized as maternal health issues, and yet, are a frequent feature in the reproductive lives of women. The high probability of poor pregnancy outcomes is not surprising, given women's poor nutritional status, overload of physical work, chronic psychological stress and intimate partner violence (Ahmadi et al. 2017; Lee et al. 2019; Qu et al. 2017; Pastor-Moreno et al. 2020).

The decision to take steps to prevent pregnancies or to stop childbearing, a fundamental reproductive right, was denied to most of the women. The experiences of women like Meenakshi with failed attempts at fertility treatment, uterine cancer, and mental health issues indicate the complexity of women's reproductive health-care needs, which often remain unmet because health systems fail women living in the margins.

Right to Essential Sexual and Reproductive Health Services

Only some of the stories contain detailed accounts of the women's need for essential sexual and reproductive health services, limiting the scope of the discussion in this section.

Health systems are vested with the express goal of ensuring basic health-care for all. Their structure, design, and functioning gives them the potential to reduce health inequities through responsiveness to the health needs of the most marginalized. Unfortunately, the Indian health system does not play such a role (Gaitonde 2018). The stories of many of the women stand testimony to this.

Pregnancy and delivery services, although widely available, eluded the women who delivered at home and lost their infants due to obstetric complications. The women's life circumstances sometimes prevented their utilization of ante-natal care, even when this was available. Some women who sought institutional deliveries, encountered obstetric violence and disrespect in the health facilities. Sarala's experience of being blamed by nurses and doctors when she arrived at the health facility on a two-wheeler, bleeding after a stillbirth, is a clear example of a health system that was insensitive to her own and her husband's disabilities.

Failure to reach girls and women with contraceptive information and services contributed to mis-timed, unwanted, and repeat pregnancies. This was the case not only in the Adivasi area of Odisha but also in urban Gujarat, Maharashtra, and Tamil Nadu, which have robust government health systems. Among the women in sex work, limited information and access to contraception resulted in repeated unwanted pregnancies and the constant fear of becoming pregnant.

For most of the women who wanted to terminate their pregnancies, safe abortion services were inaccessible or unaffordable. In the case of pre-marital pregnancies, the providers refused to provide an abortion even though the gestational period was within the legally permissible limit, which forced the women to resort to self-induced abortions using medical abortion pills, often without the necessary information; for some unfortunate women, the refusal to terminate their pregnancy could change the entire course of their lives.

Defying Victimhood: Women's Resistance and Resilience

The women in these stories may have unimaginably difficult lives but are no victims. Within their stories of severely constrained autonomy and violation of their sexual and reproductive rights, one finds embedded instances of defiance and self-determination.

Sarala, Rekha, and Sonal defied the social norm of an arranged marriage and chose their own husbands. Rekha and Sonal were ready to face the consequences of their acts of self-determination. Rukmini's decision to leave her home and continue her pregnancy at the young age of 19 years was another courageous move. Despite opposition from her mother-in-law, Sita was determined to undergo a tubectomy after her third delivery. In Vimala, Reshma, and Priya's stories of finding their feet and taking control of their lives in sex work as autonomous individuals, and in Meenakshi's amazing story of becoming a Dalit woman leader despite several challenges, one finds a resilience and the strength to surmount social and physical obstacles.

Employment and income-earning opportunities are major factors in helping these women resist oppression. As Sonal says, 'Employment increases knowledge, skill, and earnings'. She leveraged her status as an earning woman and the confidence gained at work to tackle her controlling brothers and to negotiate sexual and other decisions with her boyfriend. Deprived of parental support, Rukmini enjoys her financial independence with her meagre NGO salary and focuses on building herself. Priya felt more in control of her life after she began sex work. She practises her profession with dignity and responsibility—insists on condom use by all her customers, ensures that all her previous and current partners are regularly tested for HIV, and gets herself regularly tested for HIV. While Rekha found her work physically taxing, it provided her an escape from the daily tensions of her abusive marriage. She received good nutrition, child care, and emotional support at work, which was denied to her at home. When she was forced to resign from her job because she became pregnant after unsuccessful efforts to obtain a tubectomy, she felt that she had lost everything—her economic freedom and, along with it, her self-respect.

Many women mention the role of support systems such as natal families and local community-based organizations in enabling their resilience. In their difficult lives, these sources of support keep them going. Their narratives also mention the provision of various government/public programmes and schemes to support the vulnerable groups to which they belong. In the tribal women's stories, one learns about education schemes like the tribal girls' hostel and the scholarship for Scheduled Tribes. Government hostels for children with disabilities and a monthly disability allowance of Rs. 1,000 are support measures available for persons with disability (PwD). However, many schemes meant to support women and girls from marginalized communities are poorly designed or implemented and did not benefit the women the authors spoke with. For example, the government's adolescent girls' programmes, meant to be delivered at the community level, did not provide the girls with basic information about sexual and reproductive health.

Access to Sexual and Reproductive Justice

The preceding sections discussed the multiple and intertwined forces that shape marginalized women's access to sexual and reproductive justice based on the conceptual framework emerging from the women's stories. The framework suggests that human rights must be assured, and that equity and social justice measures must be institutionalized and practised if all women are to have access to sexual and reproductive justice.

It is contended that sexual and reproductive justice is a dynamic concept, the components of which are to be defined in a context-specific manner. Black women and women of colour feminists in the US coined the term 'reproductive justice', bringing together reproductive rights and social justice. This was a reaction to the narrow focus on contraceptive and abortion rights by mainstream feminists in the US (ACRJ 2005; Price 2010; Silliman et al. 2004). Now expanded to include the issues of other marginalized groups and hence their sexual rights, some now prefer to use the term 'sexual and reproductive justice' (Price 2010; Morison 2021).

Sexual and reproductive justice for the marginalized women represented in this book should extend beyond the four components to include the right to enabling conditions that would make possible their enjoyment of sexual and reproductive rights, ranging from access to basic needs and resources such as education and employment to decriminalization of sex work. It should also include ensuring universal access to sexual and reproductive health services, with a special focus on marginalized groups. The expanded definition of sexual and reproductive justice would, therefore, be that every person has the right to:

(a) Choose to have or not have children,
(b) Carry a wanted pregnancy to term,
(c) Choose the conditions under which to give birth or start a family,

(d) Care for their children with the necessary social support in a safe and healthy environment,
(e) Control their own body and self-expression, free from any form of sexual or reproductive oppression,
(f) Enabling conditions that would make the enjoyment of sexual and reproductive rights possible, ranging from access to basic needs and resources to changes in laws and policies,
(g) Universal access to sexual and reproductive health services, with special measures to ensure not leaving anyone behind.

REFLECTIONS ON KEY LEARNINGS AND THE WAY FORWARD

This book is an attempt at epistemic creation from below and an effort to create knowledge that will contribute to consciousness-raising among women in similar social locations, and advocacy and activism to transform these conditions.

We believe that the use of life stories has deepened and altered one's understanding of the complex forces that shape women's sexual and reproductive experiences in several ways:

- Life stories help to recognize the complex ways in which groups of people are denied sexual and reproductive justice and, simultaneously, to draw lessons for policy-making and programming from the exertion of agency by marginalized women to resisting such denial and to claiming their voices.
- Evidence on women's sexual and reproductive health usually comes in event-specific silos: menstruation, sexual interactions, pregnancy, delivery, infections, and so on. Life stories demonstrate the cumulative impact of each sexual and reproductive health event or experience on a subsequent sexual and reproductive health event or experience, and the influence of women's general health status on their sexual and reproductive health experience.

- Studies that attempt to understand the social, economic, and gender determinants of sexual and reproductive health events do not usually capture the dynamic, two-way interplay between economic and social marginalization and health, as life stories do.
- Multiple factors shape a sexual or reproductive health experience at a given point in time, which makes the experience very different for women in different social locations and amidst varying life circumstances.

In addition to the insights it has enabled, the narrative life-story method afforded room for participants to exert agency in what they chose to share, and what aspects of their sexual and reproductive lives they chose to highlight.

The emerging conceptual framework shows that it would take more than a well-designed package of sexual and reproductive health services to meet the sexual and reproductive health needs of women, especially those experiencing layers of marginalization. As civil society actors, programme implementers, researchers, and policy advocates, one needs to understand how social marginalization of different hues, nature and severity, both current and over generations, leads to the embodiment of health disadvantages and the denial of sexual and reproductive justice for marginalized women. One's actions should reflect this understanding and translate into context-specific and sensitive programme designs and agendas for advocacy, action and research.

The starting point would be to replace esoteric theorizing or mechanistic data-crunching, which do not contribute to on-ground changes, with a 'radical scholarship of praxis' (Indira 2020) that breaches the silos of academia and activism and applies itself to knowledge, co-production engaging and centring voices from the margins.

REFERENCES

ACRJ (Asian Communities for Reproductive Justice). (2005). *A New Vision for Advancing our Movement for Reproductive Health, Reproductive Rights and Reproductive Justice*. Oakland, CA: Asian Communities for Reproductive Justice.

Ahmadi, R., S. Ziaei, S. Parsay (2017). 'Association Between Nutritional Status with Spontaneous Abortion'. *International Journal of Fertility and Sterility 10*(4):337-42. doi: 10.22074/ijfs.2016.4577. Epub 1 November 2016.

Arnold, F., S. Parasuraman, P. Arokiasamy & M.T. Kothari (2009). *Nutrition in India*. 'National Family Health Survey (NFHS-3) India', 2005-6. Mumbai: International Institute for Population Sciences; Calverton, Maryland, USA: ICF Macro.

Aurino, E. (2017). 'Do Boys Eat Better than Girls in India?: Longitudinal Evidence on Dietary Diversity and Food Consumption Disparities among Children and Adolescents', *Economics & Human Biology*, 25: 99-111. doi.org/10.1016/j.ehb.2016.10.007.

Gaitonde, R. (2018). 'The Role of the Health System'. In T.K.S. Ravindran & R. Gaitonde (Eds.). *Health Inequities in India: A Synthesis of Recent Evidence*. Singapore: Springer.

Geronimus, A.T. (1992). 'The Weathering Hypothesis and the Health of African-American Women and Infants: Evidence and Speculations'. *Ethnicity & Disease*, *2*(3): 207-21.

Indira, R. (2020). 'Lending Voices to the Marginalised: The Power of Narratives as Alternative Sociological Discourse'. *Sociological Bulletin*, *69*(1): 7-16. https://doi.org/10.1177/0038022919898999

Izugbara, C. (2011). 'Poverty, Masculine Violence, and the Transformation of Men: Ethnographic Notes from Kenyan Slums'. In E. Ruspini, J. Hearn, B. Pease, & K. Pringle (Eds.) *Men and Masculinities Around the World. Global Masculinities*. New York: Palgrave Macmillan. https://doi.org/10.1057/9780230338005_17

Jewkes, R., R. Morrell, J. Hearn, E. Lundqvist, D. Blackbeard, G. Lindegger, M. Quayle, Y. Sikweyiya & L. Gottzen (2015). 'Hegemonic Masculinity: Combining Theory and Practice in Gender Interventions', *Culture Health & Sexuality*, *17*: 112-27.

Krieger, N. (2005a). 'Embodiment: A Conceptual Glossary for Epidemiology'. *Journal of Epidemiology and Community Health*, *59*(5): 350-5. doi: 10.1136/jech.2004.024562. PMID: 15831681; PMCID: PMC1733093.

Krieger, N. (2005b). *Embodying Inequality: Epidemiologic Perspectives.* Amityville: Baywood Publications.

Lee, W., S.W. Jung, Y.M. Lim, et al (2019). 'Spontaneous and Repeat Spontaneous Abortion Risk about Occupational Characteristics among Working Korean Women: A Cross-sectional Analysis of Nationally Representative data from Korea'. *BMC Public Health, 19*: 1339. https://doi.org/10.1186/s12889-019-7728-7

Morison, T. (2021). 'Reproductive Justice: A Radical Framework for Researching Sexual and Reproductive Issues in Psychology'. *Social and Personality Psychology Compass, 15*(6). doi.org/10.1111/spc3. 12605

Pastor-Moreno, G., I. Ruiz-Pérez, J. Henares-Montiel, V. Escribà-Agüir, C. Higueras-Callejón & I. Ricci-Cabello (2020). 'Intimate Partner Violence and Perinatal Health: A Systematic Review'. *British Journal of Obstetrics and Gynaecology, 127*(5): 537-47. doi: 10.1111/1471-0528.16084.

Patel, K.A., S.D. Langare, J.D. Naik & S.S. Rajderkar (2013). 'Gender Inequality and Bio-social Factors in Nutritional Status among Under-five Children Attending Anganwadis in an Urban Slum of a Town in Western Maharashtra, India'. *Journal of Research in Medical Sciences, 18*(4): 341-5.

Price, K. (2010). 'What is Reproductive Justice?: How Women of Color Activists are Redefining the Pro-choice Paradigm'. *Meridians. 10*(2): 42-65.

Qu, F., Y. Wu, Y.H. Zhu, J. Barry, T. Ding, G. Baio, R. Muscat, B.K. Todd, F.F. Wang & P.J. Hardiman (2017). 'The Association between Psychological Stress and Miscarriage: A Systematic Review and Meta-analysis'. *Scientific Reports*, 7(1):1731. doi: 10.1038/s41598-017-01792-3.

Starrs, A.M., A.C. Ezeh, G. Barker, A. Basu, J.T. Bertrand, R. Blum, A.M. Colle-Seck, A. Grover, L. Laski, M. Rao, Z.A. Sathar, L. Say, G.I. Serour, S. Singh, K. Stenberg, M. Temmerman, A. Biddlecom, A. Popinchalk, C. Summers and L.S. Ashford. (2018). 'Accelerate Progress—Sexual and Reproductive Health and Rights for All: Report of the Guttmacher-Lancet Commission'. *The Lancet*, 391(10140):2642-92.

United Nations Development Programme (UNDP) and Oxford Poverty and Human Development Initiative (OPHI). (2021). *Global Multidimensional Poverty Index 2021 Unmasking Disparities by Ethnicity, Caste and Gender* [Internet]. Available from: https://ophi.org.uk/multidimensional-poverty-index/

Contributors

ABHISHEK SEKHARAN PhD Student, School of Information, University of Michigan, Ann Arbor.

ANAGHA PRADHAN Independent consultant and researcher, Vadodara.

BIJAYALAXMI RAUTARAY Secretary, SAHAYOG, Bhubaneswar, Odisha.

MANUSHI SHETH Coordinator, Community Programmes, SAHAJ, Vadodara, Gujarat.

P. BALASUBRAMANIAN Executive Director, Rural Women's Social Education Centre, Chengalpattu, Tamil Nadu.

RENU KHANNA Founder member, SAHAJ, Vadodara, Gujarat.

SANA QAIS CONTRACTOR Independent researcher, Mumbai, Maharashtra.

SHRUTI ARORA Doctoral candidate, Queen Mary University of London.

SOUVIK PYNE Restless Development, Delhi, India.

SUBHA SRI B. Independent researcher.

T.K. SUNDARI RAVINDRAN Founder Member, Rural Women's Social Education Centre, Chengalpattu, Tamil Nadu.

TEJASWI SEVEKARI Executive Director, Saheli Sangh, Pune, Maharashtra.

V.R. ATKURI Independent public health physician.

Index